Caught in the Interstice
A Journey Through the Unseen Depths of Existence

Hailey Jeklinski

ISBN: 979-8-218-59521-0

Printed in the United States of America

Dedication

This book is dedicated to my daughter, Kalia; my husband, Tyler; my mother and father; my in-laws; my sisters, Emily and Madison; and, of course, Dr. Saxena. With continued love and support from my family, friends, and even strangers, I have made it through the deepest of trenches. I will do my best to put into words the experiences and revelations I've taken away from my battles with health over the past decade, as well as those I've struggled with since childhood. I am grateful for all those who have been part of my wild life the universe has been weaving, as well as the lessons they've presented.

And finally, this book is dedicated to you, the reader. You are not obliged to agree with or believe anything I say, though it may be in your best interest to read my words with an open mind and an open heart. We must always remain students, never assuming we truly "know" anything. This world is not what it seems – it is much, much more.

In loving memory of my PopPop, Master Sergeant Joseph "Peppy" Neluna, aka Six Pack. 2/18/50–12/28/24

"Knowing your own darkness is the best method for dealing with the darknesses of other people."

\-   Carl Jung

Contents

FOREWORD

by Tyler Jeklinski

As a 16-year-old boy, I was awestruck by the beautiful girl who frequently looked my way with her deeply mysterious and stunning brown eyes in the hallways of Southern Regional High School. Being young, I didn't know what the future might hold, but I did know one thing: this girl would be a part of my life forever. With that being said, I never expected the journey our life together would take us on.

When Hailey asked me to write the foreword for this book, I didn't know where or how to start. Having spent more than half our lives together, there was too much to fit into a few paragraphs. However, as time went on, I realized that the specific details of our life together didn't matter as much as the lessons I've learned from her as my life partner. I knew I could put my best foot forward (pun intended) to write this foreword as succinctly and impactfully as possible.

We all face some type of adversity in our lives. Whether we grow from those challenges, regardless of how difficult they are, is a choice. Some people face difficult circumstances and wallow in their struggles, while others face them with a full head of steam. Some people like to bring those around them down, while others not only better themselves in the face of adversity but also motivate those around them to become better individuals. I've been lucky to stand by someone who has faced some heavy shit. Through facing this adversity, Hailey has, time and time again, grown from these struggles, and greatly inspires those around her by doing so. Despite how she might downplay her experiences in the coming pages, I can tell you firsthand that Hailey knows how to get knocked on her ass by a freight train and get right back up. I hope this book provides you, the reader, with infinite inspiration that no matter how many times you get knocked down, no circumstance should ever keep you there.

Witnessing Hailey's journey has been my biggest blessing. It has completely changed my outlook on this trippy experience we call life and taught me things about love that take lifetimes to learn. And I don't just mean romantic love. I'm referring to the all-pervasive love that fuels this life experience. What you are about to read will take you, as it did me, through a range of emotions. Much may be relatable, and other parts might be difficult to comprehend. You are not alone in feeling that way. But if I can suggest one thing to consider when reading this book, it is to look for the lessons. Focus less on the details, and more on the big picture. I have been lucky enough to not personally go through the things Hailey has, but I have learned just as impactful lessons in my own way by witnessing her experiences and hearing her perspectives. I hope this book can do the same for you. Life is fragile and sometimes may seem unfair, but there is always a deeper meaning to the things with which we are presented. I hope the fact that you have opened this book can provide you with some variation of depth to become a better individual yourself.

Over the last seven years, I've seen this book written and rewritten countless times. Hailey would write for months on her phone, then delete it in a rage because she felt "nobody would care" or "it was just too much." I pleaded, until I was blue in the face at times, telling her she needed to get her message out there. However, I finally concluded that when she was ready, she would write her book. That time has finally come. I can't express how proud I am of her for finally sharing her experiences with the world.

To Hailey – I love you. I am so proud of how brave and courageous you are for openly sharing your story. Never stop being you. To the reader – I wish you a life full of love and presence. May this book guide you on your journey from the head to the heart.

Part 1

Echoes of Truth: Navigating the Shadows of Illness and Identity

16

PREFACE

There are books that will tell you what's "right" and "wrong", there are books that will tell you how to live, books that will give you step-by-step instructions on "how to..." – this book will not follow suit. Though I have personally been through the wringer a few times, the knowledge I've acquired cannot necessarily be taught, which is why writing this book has been so difficult. I cannot, and will not, provide you with the answers you're seeking. You are the one who holds the key to all of life's secrets that yearn to be acknowledged, just as I am the only holder of the keys of the many doors I've been lucky enough to stumble through.

We are all on our own journeys, therefore the doors I've stumbled through are for me and me only. The doors you travel through are your own, and although some paths traveled may seem similar, each one is unique as they provide deep-seated teachings that correspond to the karma and personal perception of each individual soul. The decisions we make, the encounters we engage in, and the work we're all putting into these lives we currently find ourselves in, are all vitally important to a grander whole mission.

It has taken me quite a while to even begin to understand the lessons I've collected in my current life. The diagnoses I was given and their challenges, the events leading up to them, as well as the events that followed, have all lead me down some dark, dark places. But on the other side of each dark place I've so far been to, there was light. There has always been light.

It's been challenging for me to attempt to list the lessons I've learned over the years because healing, evolving, and understanding cannot be organized with the literal mind. In true reality, nothing is linear. Time, space, experiences, healing, none of these are actually occurring in a linear sequence - all are happening simultaneously. Our minds tend to organize things to make them make more sense, but the illusion has to be recognized in order for you to break through the lessons at hand - or else it will be missed and you will have to repeat them over and over until you really "get it". Things you go through can and will be repeated over and over again, that's inevitable. What's funny about being more aware of oneself is that once you think you've finally cracked the code, or learned the lesson, the more experiences will present themselves and test you to see if you've really mastered the teaching... and this will happen for the rest of your life. In the wise words of Nahko Bear, "the work is never done".

To really digest the words in this book, please give yourself a bit of a break. You're temporarily using these bodies as vehicles to guide you to new heights in your own personal soul evolution, which extends way beyond this physical world. When you can somewhat comprehend complex topics, as much as you can within the frame of the human mind, then you're opening yourself up to a new portal of understanding. This cycle doesn't stop - you will constantly be learning further than you ever have. And this widened perspective, however far, has the ability to guide you through the rest of your experience in this lifetime. Once my mind started to expand its perspectives, things got "easier" to deal with. Hardships, as one would experience, started to not feel as difficult as they once were. I started to have more appreciation for everything in my life. I was able to look at the experiences I've encountered and see them for what they were and ponder what they were showing me, rather than fantasizing about what could have been or getting too lost in the details.

Although life seemed to become easier, the "work" part got more demanding - for good reason. It was now my responsibility to hold myself accountable for everything that my mind engages with. From the thoughts of myself to how I interact during conflicts, each action/non-action had to be carefully curated with intent. Failure to stay on track would lead to immediate consequences, and yet staying on track would also lead to immediate consequences. And after realizing the lessons within the lessons, I started to truly embody my truest expression of "me" in those moments.

It takes a lot of dedication and focus to maintain the always ever-evolving highest version of yourself, which is why I will say it again - give yourself a break. I still must remember to take my own advice more often than you'd think. You will fall back into old habits and thoughts more times than you could count, but you'll always rise again. Each time there will be more understanding. There's no reason to rush and there's no reason to be so serious, for "time" isn't *real* anyway. So, essentially, you have an infinite amount of "time" to learn the lessons, to have the experiences. To practice, practice, practice. That's what we've come to Earth to do, to experience and put ourselves up to all the tests, to feel the spectrum of emotions - which we are lucky enough to achieve through our experiences. That's what keeps us coming back. What's the fun of fitting the entire universe's knowledge into one lifetime? Enjoy the process because the latter could be entirely different.

You may not have the ability to feel and experience in the same way on the other side. So, take it one experience at a time, get comfortable in this body, allow yourself the confusion, the frustration, the hardships, the pain, the joy – all of that will inevitably lead to love. Due to comfort and level of difficulty, many will choose to walk down other roads, but those who dedicate themselves to a path back to self will be rewarded.

Looking back on my entire life and all of the experiences so far, I'm only now realizing this was all an initiation. And although I'm still young and in my early thirties, I understand and accept that this life was never meant to be normal, and I was never meant to be ordinary. The words that fill this book took a lot of letting go. It's not so much my journey that I had a hard time writing about. It was more of a fact that I needed to somehow put into words what I've taken away from the gift of living with multiple chronic illnesses along with the challenges that come along with them and make sense of it to a world that's so sensitive - which feels like an impossible feat. You may get offended, or you may not. Regardless, this book was written from the depths of my understanding and my experiences, all of which I'm still and always will be fine-tuning. It may go against what's popular, or even sound absolutely insane, but it's all true for me. I was truly caught between two worlds of completely contrasting natures, where the outside world was out of reach – leaving me confused and horrified, I somehow navigated the interstices of my reality. Enjoy – and thank you for allowing me to take up space in your mind.

Caught in the Interstice

1

SHIFTING CURRENTS

Have you ever, for even a brief moment, questioned your reality? Have you ever pondered the idea of there being more to life than what you're seeing in front of your eyes? Doing so would broaden your perspective on all situations that occur in your life, and at some point, you'll be thankful you did. My life seemed to have been at a standstill. What now seems like ages ago, in 2015, I was diagnosed with Systemic Lupus Erythematosus (SLE), and everything about my entire reality shifted in a direction I had never thought imaginable. The pain, the loss of independence, the complete loss of self, the fear, the near-death experiences, the frustration and intense anger and rage, the head-spinning realizations - have all lead me to right here, right now.

I have started this book numerous times. Throughout the process, I have deleted the many drafts and gave up completely on finishing them, and only now, about ten years later, have I finally, somewhat, been able to find the words to express my deepest thoughts in the way I would like. I've come to terms with the fact that the "journey" is never truly over, the experiences will never end, and yet life still gets more beautiful each time I make it through the intense obstacles. Just like getting stuck in a set of pounding waves not allowing you to come back up for air - this is my story.

2

THE BACKSTORY

I grew up as an athlete, starting soccer at just 3 years old. Through travel teams, a high school team, and a college team, I made soccer my number one priority. There were days where it totally murdered me, where I wanted to give up on the one thing that was keeping me sane, days where I thought I wasn't good enough - but something about it was addicting. I became the fastest amongst my teammates, the captain of my teams, and the most mentally strong young woman - and I owe that solely to this sport. The entirety of the person I've become can all be owed to soccer and its demands. I often wondered why I was so obsessed with it. I genuinely loved it more than anyone could ever imagine, and it was my only escape from the world. Life has always been difficult for me in some respect, but soccer was the only thing I had that I didn't need to use my mind for. It just came so naturally – I'd step on a field, and everything else completely melted away. There were no worries, no struggles, and no drama. It was just me, a ball, and some grass. That was all I needed. Deep down, I knew I was setting myself up for the rest of my life through soccer. That "setting up" was just not exactly how

I imagined it unfolding.

During my second year of college, I had one of the most mentally intense seasons of my life. This led me to become more consistent and stronger than I had ever been. If I had paid closer attention, I would have been able to tell that everything going on during this time was all too good to be true and was happening for some deeper reason. But what was that reason? Why would I fall so in love with a sport only to have it blindly ripped away from me? For years, I had dedicated all of my free time to perfecting this game. And soon after that amazing, heartfelt last season in college came my first diagnosis; stripping away an identity I had been strongly attached to my whole life.

3

THE LITTLE GIRL IN ME:
LEADING UP TO THE FIRST DIAGNOSIS

In the summer of 2014, my husband, Tyler, and I both came down with mononucleosis. This illness triggered an entirely new set of events within my body, and by the following winter, my body started to stop cooperating with me. Getting dressed became difficult, and every inch of my body was in constant, piercing pain. I had no idea what was going on and actually blamed myself, thinking it was because I hadn't kept up a proper off-season workout schedule after ending the previous soccer season.

My home life wasn't the greatest, but it also wasn't the worst. Verbal and physical abuse were part of my life from a young age, but I kept that pretty quiet. Like any child, I thought it was normal. Money was a luxury that my family didn't have much of. Food and heat were scarce; sometimes we had to sleep at a hotel or in our car as a family of four — but my parents always made it work. They were young, having me at only 18 and 17, with my sister being born about five years later. Having children at such an early age is challenging, especially when you're still growing up yourself. Financial stress with two children and two dogs created a chaotic environment. Constant fighting seemed like the baseline in our household, so I grew up much faster than most kids my age. I remember being home alone with my sister often when we weren't at school because my parents were working multiple jobs to keep a roof over our heads. We moved from rental to rental every few years, so I never had that "white picket fence" type of environment. As I've grown older, I've realized that was for the best, but this resulted in feeling as if I had too many responsibilities for my age.

As far back as I can remember, I've dealt with major anxiety and stress running through my body at all times. Too young to understand what those words even meant, I internalized these emotions, which caused issues that spilled into adulthood. I was always scared that my parents would fight, and I would get severe stomach aches from the anxiety, often wanting to be picked up early from school just to escape the fear. On top of this, I grew to be a light sleeper and always felt like I had to keep one ear open. Even today, I wake up to the slightest noise, always ready and alert. My dad and I had a tough time getting along, and I felt like I had to walk on eggshells around my parents, either to avoid starting a fight between them or to avoid punishment myself.

Growing up, I became very independent at an early age.

Watching my parents work so hard, doing whatever it took to get a paycheck, embedded a unique mindset in me like no other. It showed me the importance of "doing what you've got to do," so I did whatever I needed to survive. I started working at 13 and held as many jobs as my schedule would allow. If I wasn't at school or soccer, I was working. Most of my jobs ran me down to the core. Between early mornings, late nights, terrible pay, and unfair treatment, the cumulative stress took a toll on my mind and body. But of course, as I had done before, I ignored those signs.

So, if you haven't already pieced it together, I was an anxious, overworked, underpaid go-getter who felt like I had to do it all and didn't know when to stop. I constantly felt the weight of the world on my shoulders, as if everything was my responsibility. I was always go-go-go until I'd burn out, but that was the catch — I never burned out. I worked multiple jobs at once, went to college, played on two soccer teams (one for school and one travel team), managed the stress of my home life, and maintained a new relationship with a boy who is now my husband. I did all this while trying to save up enough money to buy a car, pay for college and all its expenses, and move out of my hometown. At this point in my life, my mental health was complete shit. Looking back, I understand now that I was like this because I knew that only I could provide the sense of security and independence that I needed. It wasn't the smartest approach, but at the time, I felt I had no other choice. Survival mode was the only mode I had ever known.

So, where am I going with all this seemingly unnecessary information? When you add up years of constant stress, starting from an early age, compounded by a lack of sleep due to anxiety or long work hours, plus pushing your body to its limits in pursuit of becoming a professional soccer player, eventually you *will* burn out. There's no escaping it. Everything comes to an end. This "ultra-independent, psychotic, go-getter" cycle of needing to be perfect and provide for myself ended in 2015.

4

AN INVISIBLE WAR

In June of 2015, I was diagnosed with Systemic Lupus Erythematosus. Months before the diagnosis, I'd received a flu shot in December 2014, just a short time after recovering from mononucleosis. Immediately afterward, I noticed excruciating joint pain, constant migraines, and a butterfly-shaped rash on my face that I dismissed as sun poisoning. This reaction was the last straw for my already overwhelmed immune and nervous systems. Needless to say, that was the last vaccination I ever received—but I won't get into that extremely controversial, touchy subject since everyone's so soft nowadays. You do what you feel is right for you.

At first, I honestly didn't take the lupus diagnosis too seriously. For the first couple of years, I just let it happen without giving it much focus. I dealt with the pain which I was used to by this point in my life. I tried numerous medications, none of which made a difference for the intense, all-pervasive pain I was experiencing. Frustration was piling up quickly.

Due to the fact that I was freshly 21 years old in 2016, I felt I was allowed to treat my body however I wanted. College parties and binge drinking were normalized in this phase of my life. You can ask anyone who knew me at this time, and they would all agree that Tyler and I were a truly wild pair. "Nutcases" if you will. I would tell myself the steroids I was on would counteract the consequences drinking had on my body. There was one night in particular where I decided to not give a single fuck. I was on a few different medications, steroids, and a medication that was considered a low-dose chemotherapy drug (one that you are certainly not supposed to drink alcohol while taking). I went to a pre-game party before a concert at my college and ended up in the medical tent by the end of the night. I had told myself prior that I didn't care what happened to me and had the bright idea of drinking almost an entire plastic water bottle filled with rum, after already having taken multiple shots along with smoking weed. The full details of this story are usually told in a joking manner, although it was clearly a desperate cry for help. I also have always tended to turn my trauma into humor because if I don't laugh, I'll cry. There was nothing actually funny about the deeper meaning of that entire situation though.

By the time 2017 rolled around, I had lost much of my independence by this point. My body hurt so bad every second of every day. Each time I'd drag myself out of bed to take a shower, I would just break down in uncontrollable tears. There were many times I'd talk to whatever was listening (God?): "Please take this away from me, I don't deserve this! Why is this happening? What did I do wrong?" I eventually learned that these were the wrong questions to be asking. Thinking back to those days still makes me feel unsettled because of how badly I wanted to end it all. I was in so much physical pain and was so completely lost within myself on how to mentally handle what I was experiencing. Prior to this, I was used to my body doing anything I wanted it to do, and now I was so restricted. I truly felt so alone because no one I knew really understood this type of pain at my age.

During the first couple of years of the diagnosis, since my body was declining pretty quickly, I wasn't able to start soccer back up again that season in 2015. I had to put my pride aside and realize that my body was becoming too fragile. I was absolutely devastated to say the least. How did I go from a 130-pound solid athlete to being weak and rickety, comparable to an elderly woman? I eventually was forced to make the decision to stop working because of always having to call out or go home early due to being in so much pain. Overall, I just wasn't functional. This was a huge turning point for me since all I ever prioritized was keeping myself busy and productive, so this was one of the hardest situations I needed to succumb to.

So, soccer was blindly torn away from me, and I couldn't physically hold a job anymore. What did I have left? I had spent a good chunk of time sulking and feeling sorry for myself, and I definitely was not a joy to be around. Those feelings are most definitely valid, although allowing oneself to stay in such a desperate state isn't healthy and will only speed up the process of illness. And, oh boy, did it ever. At this point, I was so miserable and depressed. I needed assistance with dressing because it hurt to lift my arms and maneuver a shirt over my head. I needed help showering, making it up and down the stairs, and most of the time I couldn't even lift a cup of water to my mouth. My joints were so inflamed everywhere, I felt like broken glass. My body felt like it was giving up on me. And this all sent me into a really dark place. What is the point of living when you feel this much pain every waking moment, along with the intense mental spiral that comes along with it? I was heading down a slippery slope.

After coming across numerous blogs (when that was still a thing), I gained some inspiration to start sharing what I was experiencing publicly. Through social media, mainly Instagram and a WordPress blog that's no longer active, I was able to put out in the public eye that I was not okay, but

I was still surviving. This drew a lot of people's attention, especially from those in a similar boat that I was in. I learned from others suffering on this path, as well as taught the little that I thought I knew. It was sort of a coping mechanism – if I shared what I was going through and someone reached out, I felt as if my experience was being validated. And that made me feel good and not so alone anymore. Starting that blog is what sparked my "healing" phase. I gained the motivation to not just give up, and to help others get out of their slump, all while still being in my own. I was able to create connections with people from all over the world. We were our own little sick support family. 2017 was when I really started to take things seriously with my health – that's when I quit my multiple jobs, began to change the way I thought, became more conscious of what I was putting in and on my body, and started being more appreciative of the life I was living. I really gave a lot of focus to shedding the old, miserable, bitchy, and sour versions of myself that I knew I was lugging around for most of my life.

If there's one thing I learned from my many years in the hole, it's that mindset is absolutely everything. That may sound so "new age", but it couldn't be closer to the truth. You cannot achieve happiness by having a miserable attitude. There was a point in my life that I was so miserable that I wanted to end it all - on more than one occasion. I couldn't take the pain, the no answers, and blank stares from doctors when I'd ask in-depth questions about my situation, or the fact that I was uncontrollably taking out my anger and frustration on the ones I loved. With the burden aspect of everything (which was the biggest killer), and the fact that I couldn't live my life like every other twenty-something-year-old, this all kept me in a resting, depressive state. I completely withdrew from the world; I didn't want anyone else to have to suffer because of my personal suffering. When you're in that deep of a hole, you hardly recognize any of the positive things that are occurring in your life and tend to only focus on all of the negative, which inevitably breeds more negative experiences.

5

A SPARK IN THE DARK

I had and still have the most amazing support system. My husband, my parents, my in-laws, and the amazing friends I had met through my blog were always there for me. My husband, Tyler, is not only my greatest supporter but also my most influential teacher. His unwavering dedication to our relationship has shaped me into the woman I am today. Without him, I genuinely don't know where I would be. He inspires me to embrace my own strength, and because of his love, I have the confidence to face any challenge that comes my way.

When I'm screaming at the top of my lungs because of a medication-induced psychotic episode, he's there. When I'm on my hands and knees during a costochondritis flare not being able to take a proper inhalation, wanting to kill myself, he's there. When I'm vomiting from a swollen stomach or medication changes, he's there. When I mentally left this earth and could no longer make decisions for myself in the hospital and had no sense of self or time, he was there – regardless of the intense rage I took out on him. This angel of a man is really here for it all, good or bad, and that knowing in and of itself is what keeps me going every day.

Watching someone you love go through such challenging health obstacles over and over again has to be the worst feeling. As someone who was sick in this relationship, I can't imagine the struggles that came along with being in the opposite position, but I do know it's far from easy. The difficulties that come along with that role cannot truly be explained in words, only experiences. I do know that what I experienced within myself during the hardest time of our life was equally experienced inside of Tyler – it just manifested itself in two separate ways. I could write an entire book on solely the appreciation and love I have for this man, and although more than deserving, that isn't what this book was supposed to be about. (However, I have been urging him to write a book on his perspective of everything we've gone through with my health and the impact it's had on our relationship, so maybe we'll see that in the future).

6

FALSE STARTS

After I started taking my health more seriously, I started to slowly see changes (emphasis on the *slowly*). Food played a huge role in lessening my symptoms, as well as working on my mindset while settling into a meditation practice. Being more aware of myself and my surroundings was the key. Originally, when I had drafted this book the first few times, I had an entire section on food, what to eat and what not to eat – but because of my experiences and constant growth throughout this "healing" process, I finally realized that there are no right answers. This realization didn't come easy though, and I had to go through some pretty major ups and downs during my diet transitions. I've been vegetarian, vegan, gluten-free – I've partook in basically all of the dietary fads. My extremely unsuccessful and hellish journey with food lasted a span of 6 years. My biggest overarching takeaway is that none of those "dietary identities" means you're healthy, which was a really difficult concept for me grasp at first. I now know that your blood type also plays a huge role in what types of foods either make you thrive or drain your soul. So, with that being said, during the obsessive food journey I had unknowingly undertaken, I learned that no diet is fit for every person. Your body changes like the seasons, and always needs to be considered in ways that fit the specific season it is in. If you were looking for advice on how to eat for your illness, you won't find it here. What's helped me and my body will not work the same for you. Eating intuitively is the closest thing to an answer I can give you. When you give enough focus to your body for so long, it finally starts to talk to you. It will always tell you what it needs and what it doesn't want. Only *you* know what your body needs to thrive, you just have to really tune in and listen to your intuition. Don't buy into anyone trying to sell you a cookie-cutter dietary fad.

What should be a no-brainer – stay away from bioengineered foods, color additives, certain oils, processed foods, processed sugar, fake meats, fast food, pesticides, and high-fructose corn syrup. (This list would be a lot longer if I cared more to tell you the horrific truth about most of the foods that are available today, but I'll let you jump down that rabbit hole on your own time). Eating a diet filled with these ingredients can lead to things like systemic inflammation, diabetes, an overactive liver, weight gain, and so much more. Take the time to look up the ingredients in your foods to see what they could be doing to your body. We live in a fast-paced world, where convenience is everything, but it might be wise to think twice before going to the drive-thru. Try to eat organic when you can and really clean your organic fruits and vegetables. No matter who I have asked, no doctor has ever recommended any type of advice on food, which is a mind-boggling concept to consider. As a society, we focus on remediation of symptoms, but never consider prevention. Also, I just want to make it clear that I am in no way giving any type of medical advice. I'm just saying, the same way you don't need a church to find your way to God, you don't always need a doctor to find your way to good health.

7

DIAGNOSIS DOMINOES:
ONE AFTER THE OTHER

When I was diagnosed with Lupus, I was subsequently diagnosed with sister diseases such as Fibromyalgia, Sjögren's syndrome, and Raynaud's syndrome in the years following. Not ending there, in 2019, I was diagnosed with a rare illness named Kikuchi-Fujimoto Disease. It's pretty confusing, but before the actual diagnosis of that, I had experienced a 6-month flare of extremely high fevers daily. Yes, daily. Kikuchi-Fujimoto is not yet a well-understood disease despite our supposed medical advancements, but what is actually known, in a noticeably brief description, is that it's a disease of the lymph nodes. However, how it manifests in each person varies from case to case. During this aforementioned flare in 2019, my joint pain came back, and my fevers never budged, ranging from 101 to 105. I was losing weight pretty quickly, especially because when high fevers are making their debut, the last thing you want to do is eat. My body couldn't even keep food down at this point. I had screwed my digestive system big time attempting to be a successful vegan for so long. So, this led to me being extremely malnourished while undergoing the biggest health scare of my life up to this point. It took multiple teams of doctors in the hospital, and a lot of push from me, to keep digging as to why I was having these fevers. Ironically, the diagnosis of Kikuchi-Fujimoto disease came on the 6-month mark of when this flare initially started.

Since I was experiencing these daily fevers for so long, my autoimmune response reacted quickly, and I was having so many different issues going on at one time. I was admitted to the hospital for 10 days after I had shown up to an infectious disease specialist appointment with a 105.5 fever. During that stay, they found out that my lungs had been bleeding. I was told that if I had not gone to the hospital when I did, my lungs would have bled out and I most likely would've died. This was also the most stressful hospital stay that lasted what felt like 10 years long. No one knew at first what was wrong with me and I was literally quarantined on the Infectious Disease floor. This whole situation was pre-Covid, so I couldn't even imagine what this experience would've been like if it was during this psychotic state of the world we are in today. Different teams of doctors constantly came into my room around the clock asking millions of questions. Many of them blamed it all on Lupus – and if it wasn't for me standing up for myself, I would've gone home thinking this was only Lupus-related. Tyler and my mom got me through that stay, as well as the women's World Cup that I watched every game of. Also, our roommate and closest of friends, Ethan, who was also a huge support of mine at this time, had brought Zion, my service dog, to the hospital to visit me frequently. In a time of such chaos, this was a very needed piece to help me get through the stress of this situation.

I left that hospital stay with some prescribed oral steroids and a Lupus Pneumonitis diagnosis on top of everything else I had going on. Prior to this, Lupus never had affected my body internally, it was always external physical ailments, but this time it was affecting my organs – which was a scary thought to bear. By the end of 2019, I got the Kikuchi-Fujimoto diagnosis after a confirmed biopsy of my lymph node. The fevers stopped and I had found myself stuck in a very mild steroid psychosis for a bit, but that came and went in a flash. This looked like stereotypical mania; absolutely no sleep, extreme organization, the need to write everything down and make lists, had to get everything prepared for the following day, aggressive outbursts, and excessive hyperactivity. Little did I know, at this point, that these side effects from the steroids were nothing compared to what was to come in 2021.

[Fun little side story - after I had gotten the biopsy of my lymph node in my armpit in New York that led to the Kikuchi-Fujimoto's diagnosis, I flew back home to Colorado shortly after. I am not sure why I was allowed to fly on a plane that soon after surgery, but I ended up getting an infection at the incision site. It was super painful, and at one point, swelled to the size of a hockey puck. I remember getting out of the shower and calling for Tyler to come check it out because my armpit was hurting more than usual. He took a look at it, and it literally exploded. It looked like milky coffee (or as Tyler refers to it, my "caramel macchiato incident"), shooting out of my armpit. I started to have an anxiety attack due to the steroids, threw a robe on, then Tyler and Ethan drove me back to the hospital. If you couldn't tell, it was just one thing after another at this time. This ironically ended the 2019 flare, and going forward, I started to recover from it all after this incident was taken care of. Shoutout to Ethan, though. Sorry for spilling my armpit on the back seat of your Santa Fe.]

8

ONE-WAY TICKET TO HELL

After that flare, Tyler and I decided to set a date for our wedding that we had been waiting for since getting engaged in 2018. We got married in Estes Park, Colorado in August of 2020, on our 10-year dating anniversary. It was the absolute best day of my life. We were surrounded by our closest friends and family in the middle of the Rocky Mountains. I felt amazing and, at that point, my health was the most stable it had been since first being diagnosed. It was such a beautiful experience filled with so much love.

By Christmas time that year, Tyler and I were newly married living in our new apartment in San Diego, California. We voluntarily moved around quite a bit during the time of my health unpredictability, which kept things light. I had made dietary changes in the earlier part of the year that aided my digestion, I had gained weight back, my hair was growing back, and I was able to be somewhat physically active again. I truly felt the healthiest I had ever been since 2015. But, of course, being the hero and always needing to take things head-on with everything I've got, I ignored my body's needs and allowed the stress from numerous life events occurring at that time to take over, which of course, led to a fever. And another fever. And another. And after about a couple of weeks of constant fevers late that November in 2020, it all really started to spiral out of control. I couldn't believe that what we thought to be another Kikuchi-Fujimoto flare was recurring. I had fevers around the clock again from November of 2020 until May of 2021. What had happened in that "short" period of time felt like a century, and this span of time was one that will never be forgotten. I just couldn't catch a break. What a way to start off our marriage, right?

I let the fevers run their course around the clock, only taking Tylenol initially, as I knew the course of treatment that would've been suggested first was steroids. This was a treatment I wanted to avoid at all costs. My days were spent lying on the couch and walking to the bathroom, as that was all the energy I was able to muster up. I barely ate any food because my stomach was so uneasy from having really high fevers. Eventually, a couple of weeks or so into this recurring flare, I reached out to my rheumatologist in New York and told him what was going on, on top of my already terrible blood work results.

Back in August of 2019, I had gotten one full round of an infused medication called Rituximab. This medicine initially seemed to calm down the fevers and other symptoms I was dealing with during the first intense flare for a short time. Rituximab is a monoclonal antibody that attaches to the CD20 protein on the surface of B-cells and some cancer cells. This helps the immune system destroy cancer cells. Although I didn't have cancer, it's commonly used for Lupus flares due to the interaction with B-cells.

When the symptoms resurfaced in 2020, our plan was to get another round of Rituximab. This is dosed between two 6-hour infusions. In February of 2021, a few months into this new flare, Tyler took me to my first round. That following week, I went for the second round. The first round went very well, and I even had the only seat in the entire clinic right in front of a giant window with a pleasant view. Since it went so smoothly the first time, it wasn't even a thought that the second round would be anything but a breeze.

On our way to the second round of the infusion, it was a cloudy and rainy day. We were driving north on interstate 5 from downtown San Diego and were greeted by a full and vibrant rainbow ahead of us on the highway. I took this as a sign that everything was going to be all right. When I got to the clinic, we waited for about 30 minutes past my appointment time until they were able to take me. This was the first sign that things started to shift with this day, despite the optimistic start. The nurse took us back, hooked me up to an IV and started to give me the pre-medications prior to the Rituximab infusion. I was given a high dose of IV steroids and IV Benadryl. When they hooked up the Rituximab, about 10 minutes passed by, when I began to notice I was becoming really itchy. I thought nothing of it at first because skin rashes were common with my flares. Then, I started to notice the itching was becoming unbearable, all while my throat started to feel tight and it was getting difficult to breathe. The nurses rushed over with a crash cart, immediately stopped the infusion, and pumped my IV with 200mg of steroids, two more doses of Tylenol, a dose of Motrin, Demerol, Ativan, three doses of Benadryl, and Pepcid. Also, this was all happening with me running a 105-degree fever. I was terrified. Steroids also exaggerate situations, so I immediately started having an anxiety attack during this whole ordeal. Tyler told me after the fact that my face turned purple, my lips turned white, and there were red circles around both of my eyes. I obviously couldn't finish the infusion, so once they got me back to baseline after what seemed like hours later, I was able to go home. I am convinced this was the moment I started to mentally lose touch with myself and with reality due to the fact I was pumped up with such a smorgasbord of drugs at one time to prevent me from getting taken down by an allergic reaction.

Following this event, it was a hard pill for me to swallow that the medication, Rituximab, which helped me the last time around, was unable to be pursued any further. My only option at this point was to agree on going back on steroids. I started my course of steroids on 10 milligrams, and ended up on 55 milligrams of prednisone in the months following. Unfortunately, it was too late in the flare, and steroids weren't helping. My fevers were still spiking up to 105 degrees consistently, with little to no breaks in between. The second the Tylenol kicked in, my fever would reduce only a tiny bit, if at all. Nothing helped. I started losing even more weight, and soon noticed I was swimming in all of my clothes. 85lbs – I was devastated that this was happening again. I was depressed for a short while this time around, and then eventually I fully mentally checked out. I then let life take me for one of the most fucked up rides it could've put me on.

Somewhere along the way, I allowed myself to be in autopilot mode. This time around was much different than 2019. I experienced anger and rage with steroids then as well, but this was otherworldly, and this dose was way higher for my even tinier body. Everything had infuriated me and I couldn't hide it. I had absolutely zero control of my thoughts or actions. I'd lash out at Tyler and whoever I interacted with. The worst part about this time was that I was aware of all of the ways I had been, but I truly had lost control, and was just a bystander in my own mind, watching this all unfold.

I was declining fast, and after discussing options with my doctor, we decided to make a trip back to New Jersey to be closer to our family. We had figured I'd eventually need to be admitted to the hospital that he worked at, so it made sense to be closer to care I was familiar with on the east coast. I somehow flew to New Jersey by myself. No one realized, not even me, that psychosis had already started or at least was as bad as it was at this point.

9

THE BREAK

The first two weeks I spent at my parents' house while Tyler was still in California are still really foggy and choppy. Like trying to remember a dream, I only remember bits and pieces, but I had this overwhelming sense of being very hyper. Talking to people was exciting, and I spoke super fast. I wasn't able to control that at all, and I found myself apologizing when I thought I wasn't making sense. There were neurological symptoms happening around this time as well that had begun in California, right before I left for New Jersey. In the middle of my sentences, my mouth would sort of twitch and droop, and my words would jumble together. I was aware of it but couldn't stop it from happening. As time went on, these symptoms kept worsening.

I was at my in-laws' house for dinner one night. I was holding a cup, trying to drink from a straw, but my drink was empty, and I couldn't stop sucking through the straw. I couldn't move my body, talk, or make any noises. I remember hearing my mother-in-law say my name, which made me aware of what was going on, but I was completely stuck and frozen in my tracks. Episodes of that catatonic state only worsened as the flare went on. I later found out that these were short absence seizures.

During those first two weeks I was in New Jersey, Tyler was still in San Diego selling all of our belongings and clearing out our apartment. Around this time was the first episode that truly showed the people around me that I was bordering on a psychotic break.

At our apartment in San Diego, we had previously been having a lot of beef with our downstairs neighbors prior to me leaving for New Jersey. They were a younger couple, and they would sit on their couch in the apartment below us in complete silence while looking at their phones. This was every single day and night. We would see inside their unit when coming down our stairs, so I can truly confirm this was the extent of their day-to-day activities. If you choose to spend your time like this in an apartment complex, of course you're going to hear every noise coming from upstairs. So, they ended up sending in multiple complaints to property management about how loud we were doing the most basic things like walking or playing with our dog. We kept getting letters from management informing us about these complaints. Crazy Hailey, in all her well-hidden psychotic rage, decided to write a very strongly worded letter to our downstairs neighbors. To spare myself from the embarrassment, let's just say it was easy to see that this letter was written by someone who was completely out of their mind.

Because of the back and forth with our neighbors, and the really intriguing letter I decided to write, I stirred the pot a little too much. The day that Tyler left our apartment for the last time, we had gotten a package in the mail. It was a small cardboard tube with no return address. Having no clue what it was, Tyler opened it, and glitter exploded everywhere, all over him and our dog. Although this was hilarious and totally something I would have done if the tables were turned, in the moment, he was furious and ended up getting into a yelling match with our downstairs neighbors.

Eventually, leaving the glitter behind, Tyler made his way across the country with our dog and the rest of our belongings. I can't recall the moment he arrived at my parents' house, but apparently, I wasn't happy to see him and was in full-blown psychosis by this point. Now, I was completely gone.

10

LET THE GAMES BEGIN

On the second day after Tyler arrived, I was getting frustrated with everyone while sitting at the dinner table, trying to figure out when we would make the trip to NYU Langone to get me admitted and try to corral these fevers. This admittance was already pre-planned with my doctor. My family wanted me to go that night, but I wanted to go the following morning. I wanted my very specific items prior to being admitted, one of them being a specific brand of organic orange juice that only a store 40 minutes away had in stock. I told Tyler and my dad to go to the store to get it for me, then decided to angrily remove myself from the conversation and go take a shower.

Once in the bathroom, I felt agitation and anger rising in my body. Standing in the shower, I decided to shave, since I knew the upcoming days would be spent in a hospital room where this would be inconvenient. While shaving, I suddenly started to feel a hot rush in my body, and my arms began shaking uncontrollably. I felt that shaky sensation creep down from my arms, all the way to my legs, and before I could even realize what was happening, my right arm raised to my chest on its own, leaving me so confused as to why this was happening. My right hand curled up, and I collapsed to the floor. It was at this time I had my first ever grand mal seizure.

What's fascinating about this situation is that I was aware of everything while this was happening to me. The second I collapsed, and my back hit the porcelain of my parents' bathroom tub, I came out of my body and watched myself have a full-blown seizure from the top of the shower. Many people don't believe in out-of-body experiences, but there's no way in hell I could ignore the fact that I was staring at my entire body from some sort of elevated perspective. I saw in vivid detail the look on my face, the blank look in my eyes, my clenched teeth, my scrunched arms, and my stiff legs. I heard all of the noises I was making. I could see the details of the bathroom as well. I saw my mother and mother-in-law run into the bathroom, finding me on the ground of the shower. The fear on their faces is a sight I'll never be able to remove from my memory. Apparently, the seizure lasted about 3 minutes, which I'm sure felt like a lifetime to those around me.

The sensations I felt while floating above my body that was lying at the bottom of the tub are tough to put into words. It was as if my face was different, but at the same time I knew I didn't have a face. Do you know how you're used to what your face feels like because it's your face? I didn't feel the face I had been used to for 26 years. It was an identity with which I was unfamiliar. I remember feeling noticeably light, pain-free, and quick. Like I could move anywhere at the speed of light. I couldn't feel the temperature of the room, and instead it felt like I was a part of the space around me. It felt as if I were being held up by something, like I didn't need to put any effort into floating, kind of like how smoke rises and settles in the air.

11

DANCING ON THE EDGE

The most impactful moment of this experience was the decision with which I was presented. While above my body, I had this intense feeling of having a choice to zoom away from my body or go back into my body. This wasn't a question that was actually asked by someone, it was more of a decision I knew within that I needed to make. Without any mind-directed thought, I chose to lower whatever form I was in, back into my body. I knew I didn't have to make that choice though, and that I had the choice to leave in that moment. Clearly, I chose to stay because I knew this life wasn't supposed to be over yet (Or so I thought).

As my physical body and non-physical awareness melted back into one, I found myself lying on the floor with my eyes open, but I couldn't speak yet. I felt completely blissful at this point. No thoughts at all, just observing. My breath was slow. My body itself was so confused, but my awareness was sharp as a tack, like I was in full observer mode. Everything and everyone around me were so chaotic, but I felt at peace. One of the worst memories to think of that never gets easier is the look on Tyler's face once I eventually was aware enough to notice he was there. I saw a glimpse of him in the doorway of the bathroom, and I remember staring into his eyes. The overwhelming fear I could feel coming from him is an eerie feeling I wish I could forget.

The EMTs took me from the bathroom and out to the ambulance. I knew what was happening, and I didn't want to go to the hospital, especially not in South Jersey of all places. The entire situation was laden with fear from everyone around me. Although fear predominated, for some reason, even though I had just had a seizure for the first time in my life, I wasn't scared. Internally, I felt calm. But what was happening with me on the outside that everyone was seeing was the opposite. It was like the inner awareness that was calm was in the background, while the steroid-raging beast on the outside was in charge of the show.

12

HOSPITAL HOPPING

[Another fun little side story! Apparently, one of the EMTs that was there helping me during my episode was extremely rude and argued with Tyler when we arrived at the hospital. This was during the Covid-19 pandemic era, and supposedly she told him he was able to come inside the hospital with me when we arrived via ambulance. When we got there, she told him he couldn't come in with me, despite reassuring him numerous times on the ride over that he could, and then started getting aggressive when he began getting upset about that fact. She ended up charging Tyler like she was going to hit him, and Tyler, being in that state, was ready to take her on. Thankfully, my mom had stepped in, held him back, and snapped him out of it so we could proceed with the night. We all still laugh about that lady and her terrible ability to read a situation to this day. I really hope she's still not out there trying to fight distressed family members.]

Due to Covid-19 restrictions, my family had to wait outside of the hospital while I was inside. The ambulance took me to a hospital in Toms River, New Jersey, which has a reputation that isn't exactly top notch. Although my mind was sharp, relaying my thoughts aloud just wasn't working out. The staff at this hospital knew I wanted to be transferred to NYU Medical Center in Manhattan, but what I was trying to say were not the actual words coming out of my mouth. I was trying to convey to them to let me leave this hospital, go in the car with my family, and we would organize a police escort to get us up to New York City quickly. This was not a plan that was actually spoken about with my family, but my overtaken steroid mind thought it was something that sounded like a fine idea at the time.

Hearing this nonsense coming from the mouth of an individual who had just had a neurological event and was alone with no one to speak for her, the experienced healthcare professionals, for some reason, took my words as truth without confirming this plan with any of my family members. So, instead of providing me with the care I needed and then discharging me, I sat there for hours alone in this hospital. My family was still outside in the parking lot, with my care team under the assumption that we were waiting for a police escort to arrive, led by a D.A.R.E. officer from my high school. I'm also quite sure the said 'officer' had been retired for almost a decade too. Anyway, I eventually escaped this hospital, of course not without some choice words to the staff from my family. Then, my father-in-law drove us all to NYU Medical Center. As I was waiting with my mom in the triage room at NYU, a second seizure happened.

I do remember bits and pieces of what was happening before the seizure, but the gaps were filled in by my family. I was hooked up to an IV when I was first admitted to NYU Medical Center, and the fluids they had started me off with were finished. Once the bag was empty, I remember looking at my mom and laughing, saying, 'That went really quick.' My mom said jokingly, 'Did it make you feel strong?' I put my arms up to flex on her, and then I started seizing again. My mom told me that I said to her, 'It's happening,' right before I had the second seizure. This seizure was different from the first and only seemed to involve my lower body, although I still ended up ripping out my IV and everything that was attached to my arms. This seizure lasted for a few minutes like the first one, except after this one was through, my brain had decided it had been through enough, and I entered a comatose state.

I was unconscious and drugged up for three days following that second seizure. Tyler and my mom sat in a chair next to me the entire time. They pumped me with a plethora of medications every day, plus I was so deep in psychosis that I was unconscious for a lot of the stay after that. I was non-verbal for about 3 days, and this was the point of my stay where my care team wasn't sure if I was going to make it. They told Tyler that they couldn't guarantee I would come out of this comatose state, especially since they weren't sure of the source of my seizures or other neurological symptoms. After a few days of a vegetative state, I slowly began showing positive signs.

This was where my perception of the outside world started to creep back in, although the parts I do remember are still fuzzy in my mind. I looked like a zombie. My eyes would barely stay open. I remember wanting to talk so much, but I couldn't even mumble. I can still see flashes of doctors funneling in and out of the room, particularly my rheumatologist coming to see me and to talk to the team of doctors caring for me. My husband had to make so many life-changing decisions on my behalf during all of this (and clearly did an amazing job, because I'm still alive to tell the story). I was in the ICU for 7 days, and after many rounds of infusions and other high-dose medications, I began to stabilize. I ended up staying in the hospital for a few days after the week in the ICU for monitoring. They ended up diagnosing me at this time with Lupus Cerebritis, which basically meant the systemic inflammation had attacked my brain. This is why the neurological symptoms were present for as long as they were.

There was nothing easy about being in the hospital for as long as I was. I was barely conscious and had to use a bedpan to shit in. Nurses, both male and female, only a couple of years older than me, had to wipe my ass. I don't think I left that bed more than once near the end of my stay. I physically couldn't. I was so weak and was now about 80 lbs. I have glimpses of them putting electrodes on my head to monitor any more seizures and some memories of Tyler and my mom being there, but those moments are barely clear or linear. I apparently made crazy requests for things I needed that Tyler had to run all over New York City to get for me. I remember the intense fear I had inside of me that I couldn't verbalize. When I left the hospital, something just didn't feel right. I remember being so angry the day I was allowed to leave knowing that I wasn't Hailey anymore. She was gone. Long gone.

13

UNINTENDED DESCENT

The entire months of April and May following my hospital stay were intense and filled with the most horrifying internal experiences I've ever faced. When I was discharged from the hospital, I was prescribed a seizure medication named Keppra and an unheard-of dose of oral steroids for my weight at the time. The number of steroids one can handle is based on their weight. I weighed 80lbs, give or take, and I was taking fifty-five milligrams of prednisone at that time. This dose was way too high for my tiny and frail body. I was already weeks into this steroid-fueled psychosis trip, which started once I hit forty milligrams of prednisone prior to my seizures. On top of the bump in steroid dosage, my mental state was exacerbated by the seizure medications I was also taking. The side effects of this medication concoction fueled a state of internal intensity, staleness, and a fear-filled, demonic perception.

This stretch of time was the hardest period of my life to make it through. I was basically letting the devil live through me. I was mentally aware though of every single thing happening in my environment, but I was having constant hallucinations which took place both internally and externally. They completely took over whoever was in the room with me. So, in the "real," outside reality, people were just seeing me as a psychotic, raging demon. Inside my personal reality, I was fending off actual demons who took over the bodies of the people who were around me. They looked and talked like my parents, Tyler, my in-laws, my sister, my friends, and the nurses who did my blood work—but in my world, they weren't really those people I knew. These 'beings' were demons (or whatever you want to call them), acting as people I knew, taunting me and driving me absolutely insane. I still get chills at the thought of how unnerving their mannerisms were. Making eye contact with them felt eerily hypnotizing, so I avoided it as much as I could.

Splitting time between staying at Tyler's parents' house and my parents' house, every day seemed to blend together. To be honest, it wasn't until recently (I'm writing this almost three years later) that I realized I was reliving the same couple of days over and over again. Imagine reliving the same couple of days over and over again for a month straight. Everything was so distorted. My memory is so jumbled from this time that I'm still working through this trauma with Tyler. It's very apparent that what I experienced during this time was not truly happening in the world of those around me who weren't in psychosis. In a way, this isn't fair to them, because I have no memory of anyone actually being there for me. I thought I was alone. My hallucination versions of everyone made it seem like they were all against me and wanted nothing to do with me. Having incredibly detailed and emotion-filled memories of things that didn't actually happen has really complicated my life, my mind, my healing, and my relationships with those I care about.

14

WHISPERS OF THE MIND

In the midst of this stretch, when I'd wake up for the day, everything felt sped up. I'd get out of bed, and somehow find myself in the kitchen either taking my medications that Tyler set out for me or eating breakfast. The time from when I'd walk downstairs to go to the kitchen didn't exist. It's like someone had a remote control that they clicked "fast forward" on the moment I got out of bed and then hit "play" when I got to the kitchen. Every part of my day was like this and there were so many gaps where I didn't know how I ended up in certain places. I'd be taking my medication, and then all of a sudden, I'd be going to the bathroom upstairs. Then, I'd go from being in the bathroom to waking up again the next day in completely different clothes, with no recollection or explanation of how (or if) the previous day ended.

At one point, I found myself sitting on the couch attempting to watch television. I kept looking at the clock on the cable box and would watch the time go backwards. It would be 1:30 in the afternoon, and I'd visually observe it travel backwards to 1:15. When I realized that wasn't normal, I'd stare at the clock to see if it would keep happening. However, once I became aware of the anomaly, time stopped. The clock never changed from 1:15.

Just like when you're dreaming and scenes change so seamlessly, I went from staring at this clock to sitting at the dinner table with Tyler's family. A consistent part of my hallucinations was the repetition of what others were saying. During this dinner, John, my father-in-law, who had been at work all day, had asked me how my day was. Then, he'd ask me again. And again. And again. And again. It had seemed never-ending. Hearing someone ask the same question over and over would irritate and piss off anyone, psychotic or not. So, my anger and frustration at this situation welled up and came out as a very offensive and emotion-filled response. To me, I had answered him all nine hundred times he had asked, and I was fed up with hearing him ask me so many times. But to him, I had only answered once, and that answer was really cruel.

Although it was dinnertime and getting dark outside, my mind changed the scene once more, and I found myself walking at the park up the street in broad daylight with Tyler. I remember my surroundings felt eerie, like something was off. While we were on the walk, I was trying to hold his hand, and he kept refusing it. He grabbed me by the wrist and pushed me away, leaving me there at the park by myself.

Once I started to feel the emotional consequence of that encounter, feeling the anxiety, stress, and rejection fill up every part of my body, the scene changed, and it was bedtime yet again.

Instead of going to bed, I was guided by this external force of sorts that seemed to control how my hallucinations unfolded, and was 'told' to sit on the chair next to the bed. So, I proceeded to sit in that same chair with my eyes closed, rocking back and forth for hours. My awareness of life was in and out, but I was fully aware of what I was physically doing. Tyler sat up in bed and tried to convince me to come lay down, but I heard voices telling me that I wasn't allowed to move from that chair. Feeling like my life depended on it, I listened to the voices. I felt like I was overtaken, but somehow was able to witness myself having a conversation with Tyler where I tried convincing him he was being the crazy one (psychotic 'God complex' at its finest). It was in this very situation that it hit me that something was wrong with me. Whatever had control over me also had control over my words and spoke for me, with my awareness watching in the background, confused at why I was talking that way. Tyler, seeming so upset and defeated, was trying to persuade this possessed version of me to come to bed. I'm not sure how this night ended.

There seemed to be a theme with these hallucinations. Everyone who I interacted with always seemed so angry and impatient with me. After talking through my experiences with Tyler after this flare, he assured me that day at the park never actually happened. I rarely left the house other than to switch back and forth between my in-laws and my parents' house.

The hallucinations that happened when I'd be at my parents' house were more intense. In my mind, my parents always seemed so angered and impatient with me. They would ignore me when I spoke to them, only giving me dirty looks that felt piercing. Due to the history I had with my family, my hallucinations took advantage of all the pent-up hurt and pain and used them against me in an intense manner. When I tried going to sleep, the hallucinations also presented in my dreams, and my dreams were no different than the day I had experienced. It felt like I was dreaming a dream within a dream, within another dream. It was all on an endless loop. Before bed, I'd take my nighttime medications, then fall asleep. When my perception would begin again within my dream, I'd be taking my medications again, then I'd go to sleep again. This happened dozens of times in one night. In my dream of me taking my medicine and falling asleep, I realized I was taking so much medication over and over again that I thought my parents were trying to make me overdose. I sobbed and screamed in terror within my dreams, and never knew when I was awake or if I was still dreaming.

At some point, I eventually woke up for the next day. I had to get blood work done weekly to check how certain markers were looking, and this particular morning, my mom took me to the lab. I was so terrified of my hallucinations at this point that I showed up to the lab wearing noise-cancelling headphones and a blindfold to block out everything and everyone, because whoever I encountered at this time would be taken over by these demonic hallucinations. The repetition took over during this appointment, and I felt like I was getting my blood drawn for days. I just wanted it to stop. This was a lab in my small hometown in New Jersey, and there had to have been people in that waiting room who knew me. I was beyond embarrassed on the inside, but knew there wasn't much else I could do to control these things.

Once all of the blood was fully drained from my body and I had to sit through the nurse's annoying, repetitive conversation, I found myself sitting at the kitchen table at my parents' house with my family sitting around me again. My sister had come over that night to show me a get-well booklet her students had made for me. I sat there while my sister sat across from me, and my mom and dad to the right of me. Apparently, Tyler was there too, which I still don't remember on my own. Somewhere during this exchange, I snapped, and like a dream, the scene changed in the blink of an eye, and I was lying on the bed in the guest room. My eyes were closed, and I was screaming and freaking out. Tyler later told me that right before this happened, I suddenly started staring straight ahead and uttered "it's happening again." Clearly, there was always a small aspect of me who was aware of what was going on, and always at the perfect time was able to communicate with the outside world for just a small moment.

This was the night I had basically completely given up. I couldn't keep playing along with the hallucinations and repetition anymore. Up until now, I had been playing along so they wouldn't get "mad" at me, as they were constantly taunting me if I tried fighting back. By this point, I had no more energy for it. Tyler, my parents, and my sister were all surrounding me near the bed. I had asked aloud for them all to hug me so I would know they were real. In their reality, they were all hugging me together, but what I was experiencing was them standing at the end of the bed by the closet, staring at me with taunting looks on their faces, not saying any words or moving. I remember telling them that I couldn't see or feel them hugging me, but I still got no reaction from the line of people I was looking at.

This scenario was a huge turning point in the flare. It was in the middle of the night, and Tyler ended up calling my doctor to explain what was going on. Not knowing how to move forward, Tyler made the ultimate decision to try to get me to go to sleep, hoping I'd be better by the morning. They all knew that taking me to the hospital would've ended with me being admitted to a psych ward, which most definitely would've killed me. After that night, we started to slowly taper off the high-dose steroids that I had been on for months.

On a side note, Tyler recorded some of that night on his phone so that he could show my doctor the severity of my state of mind. It wasn't until over a year later that we had the courage to watch it. I was able to explain to Tyler in more detail what was happening in my reality as they watched me fade further into psychosis. There was a point in the video where my mom tried to touch my arm, and I screamed for her not to touch me. In my world, it was a hallucination version of her taunting me with a scarily seductive smirk on its face, and I didn't want it near me. However, in their reality, it was just my mom trying to comfort me. Comfort that I desperately needed, but the distorted perception I was faced with wouldn't allow me to comprehend that my family was always attempting to help me.

15

AGAINST THE CURRENT

From when the tapering of the steroids started, it took a couple of weeks for the severity of my hallucinations to ease up. Going from fifty-five milligrams to zero milligrams of steroids takes a long time, as tapering too fast could have caused more issues. At some point during the taper, my dad had taken me out for the day since I seemed to be getting a little less psychotic. We had planned to go to lunch near the beach. On our way to the beach, I had to use the bathroom, so we stopped at a CVS along the way. Still being in psychosis, my mind made me see this bathroom as the most disgusting place I'd ever stepped foot in. This was also during Covid, so in my steroid-filled mind, I was terrified of getting sicker. The hallucinated dirtiness of the bathroom set off a tantrum of sorts, and as this was happening, my dad locked me in the bathroom alone with the lights off (he didn't actually do this, this was just what my mind turned this situation into). Being in the "dark" triggered voices, and the external force that was in charge of my hallucinations surrounded me in all directions. I was so scared. When that finally ended, I found myself stumbling out of CVS with my dad guiding me down the aisles to the exit, as I screamed at all the employees for keeping such a dirty environment. Fortunately, this is one of the last really bad hallucinations I had experienced, as I continued to taper off the steroids.

During this time, there were many unsettling feelings that stick with me to this day. I always felt so alone and on guard, like I had to watch over my shoulder at every moment. My perception made me feel like everyone around me was talking about me or laughing at me. I was so scared to close my eyes to go to sleep, even after the steroids were finished. I would lay my pajamas out or put my pillow somewhere specific, and when I'd go to use those things, they'd be back in their original spot. It would infuriate me because I thought the hallucinations were messing with me and undoing things I wanted done. I wasn't allowed to have an ounce of control. I desperately just wanted to be held tightly and told that I was going to be okay. I just wanted a fucking hug, which I'm sure I got a lot of throughout my flare, but my mind blocked me from seeing or feeling this part of the support I had.

At some point during the tapering of the steroids, I had finally come to the realization that I was hallucinating, so I started attempting to pay attention as much as I could. I picked up on patterns, and I'd notice that they wouldn't get triggered if I did routine things in different locations. For example, instead of taking my medications in the kitchen,

I'd take them in the living room, or in the dining room. I did this for a while, although eventually I ran out of places to use. If I repeated the same motions from the previous days, even slightly, my reality would cross with the hallucination world, and it wouldn't end until the following day. Sometimes I'd try to secretly record on my phone the interactions I'd have with my family so I could go back and listen to see if what I remembered had actually happened. I never remembered to go back and listen to them. Sometimes the hallucinations lasted days at a time. How my mind was able to formulate these weird but clever ways of coping to help me in getting through this is beyond me. Eventually, as the steroid dose got lower, they happened a lot less often and I started to see things for what they really were.

16

AWAKENING FROM THE ABYSS

If you've ever had the opportunity to experience a psychedelic trip, my 3-and-a-half-week hallucination fiasco was comparable to a demonic nightmare of a trip. I was stuck in a false reality, where constant loops replayed themselves over and over again. I wasn't able to escape a stale environment filled with horrifying and sickening encounters. I felt so incredibly helpless. I had convinced myself numerous times throughout this experience that I had died, and I was stuck in hell. My hallucinations had played along with that thought process too, which made things a lot worse. They also would tell me that if I were to kill myself, then I'd be stuck in their world forever, which must've been my mind's clever way of keeping me alive. I am still not sure where I was mentally during this time, but I was most definitely not in my normal base reality on earth in this body. I was just silently watching from a deeper part of my own hidden universe the entire time.

Although I was slowly coming to, tapering off the steroids in and of itself was a tough level to endure. I was gradually coming back into a more conscious reality, but I wasn't fully accepting of this familiar place yet. Instead, I was constantly teetering between two different worlds. I know there were worried friends who wanted to see me, but I was too scared of everyone because I didn't know who exactly I'd be seeing, so I refused to meet with them. I couldn't tell who or what was real or fake. This bouncing back and forth between true reality and the hallucination realm lasted a pretty long time, even post-steroids.

The more linear time trickled by after fully tapering off the steroids, the more I mentally came back into perceiving this reality. When this flare first started, we had planned to move to Hawaii later that year. We stuck to this plan, despite the chaos. When I became more stable, Tyler left for Hawaii to get our new life started. He had already been in Hawaii for a month before I arrived there, trying to get us settled in our new home state by finding us a place to live before he started his new job. I hated that he went without me, and I felt like I was left behind, having to literally force my way out of New Jersey to get back to my husband. By the time I eventually got there, I wasn't even close to being fully better. I made it seem like I was, but I was still experiencing hallucinations, and they were very much present in my everyday interactions. However, this time around, I had at least one foot in this reality, so they weren't able to control me nearly as much. I didn't tell anyone this was still going on, and even Tyler only found out about it a year later.

I've realized that, for me, psychosis was like diving to the bottom of the ocean. I couldn't just come up for air, I had to first swim up level after level before being able to make it to the surface, or the "real world." As mentioned above, I wasn't fully back to the surface for quite a while, although it might have seemed that way from the outside looking in. So, when I arrived in Hawaii, the next phase of this seemingly never-ending flare had only just begun. I knew I wasn't showing up as the Hailey I had been before the flare. Tyler and I were away from each other for almost a month, with little communication. I didn't know if he was going to like who was showing up, let alone know if I was going to be meeting the same Tyler I had known since I was 15 years old. I was numb in a sense, but I knew I was alive. I had no emotions and no idling thoughts, I just existed. When this new life began, beyond devastated, I came to realize that we were now two complete strangers living in the same house.

17

END SCENE: FINAL WORDS

Finding words to explain everything seems impossible, but I've tried my best to explain my experiences and put the pieces together in a way that could be understood. I still feel like I can't make sense of all of my experiences in the linear way I would like to, so it's understandable if you are still a little confused when trying to relate to what I had experienced. There is such a disconnect between what I was experiencing and what actually happened, but what I had described above was from my point of view. Tyler has filled in a lot of the gaps of perception for me in great detail, and I'm very aware that this will be an experience that will take a long time to fully unpack on an emotional level. Given my experience, I'm confident that there's an offshoot reality parallel to this one, where a version of myself is experiencing her reality in the same way I did during psychosis, caught in the hellish interstice for eternity. I'm so grateful that this current version of me was fortunate enough to escape when she did.

Although this was the toughest and scariest experience of my life so far, I've learned more about myself and the human experience in this 3-dimensional world we live in than ever before. I have yet to be able to find the words to expand on my perception of life now, but I do understand that the way I take in information, think, and process things is truly a gift. If the experiences in my life had not played out this way, I wouldn't be where I am or who I am today. I also have a passionate trust in the universe. I trust fully in all things, which in my opinion, was the entire point of everything that happened. For those who operate on a more logical, material, or factual level, I know this must seem absurd.

I've realized after drafting this book a million times, that the nitty-gritty details were never supposed to be the point of this experience (as is true for all experiences after all). Everything unfolded in the way it should have. What matters most is that I take the lessons learned and the information available to me now and apply them to my life so that I can continue to reach new levels as an evolving soul. I will not take this life for granted, because who knows how many lifetimes it has taken me to get to this point. And whether or not you believe in other timelines, dimensions, or realities, it's difficult for me to deny the fact that I was living in separate worlds, simultaneously. This is something I would not wish upon my worst enemy. To save your own sanity from trying to follow along on a road of the darkest of thoughts, this concludes the story portion of my journey. The rest of this book will include the insights I have acquired while being in an altered state, along with lessons I've learned throughout my life. Sick or healthy, I intend for the lessons I've dissected to benefit you in some way. Remember not to take the following so literally. Sometimes the real lesson lies within the pauses, deep within the silence.

Part 2

Wisdom Woven in Fire: A Tapestry of Life's Insights

PREFACE

I personally am not one to dwell on the details, although we can't ignore that they make for a juicy story. In reality, the details never truly matter. As human beings, we are drawn to dramatize things, either for our own benefit or to fill some type of attention-seeking motive, and that can lead you down a very self-destructive road. If you take a second to look beyond that, you'll see that the stress that caused the illness, the illness itself, the circumstances, the degree, the job, the status, the "story," the "he said, she said"—none of that matters in the grand scheme of life. What's profoundly important here is what is learned and applied from the challenges you face. Oftentimes, you'll be tested over and over to see if you'll apply what you've learned. When you fail to see the lesson for what it is or fail to implement that learned lesson into your life, you'll again find yourself in a situation of similar nature—until you really "get it.

One of two things will happen at this point; you'll either recognize the repeating lesson and take action using your newly acquired realizations; or you'll fall into the trap of reacting in a similar way as you've done in the past that failed to lead you to your most desired outcome. You cannot escape, but you can choose how you react. You'll always have the choice to choose how you want to respond to any situation.

At the end of my flare in 2021, I had the choice to fall victim and ride that familiar wave like I had the first time around in 2019, or I could somehow implement all that I had learned from these experiences. One of those options would lead me to a whole new life, while the other would have kept me trapped in this cycle of illness. Fortunately, I chose an option I never had considered before, even though it was technically the "harder" path. I chose to embrace the scariness and uncomfortable ways of this unknown new perception I had gained, regardless of the fact that those around me weren't accepting of it at first.

***

A difficult part of pain and suffering in any form is the inevitable emotional attachment that we grow to have to that state of being. It's not easy attempting to disconnect from that extremely tight cord. We get so used to that familiar feeling, and in a twisted way, it actually makes us feel safe. But it's a false sense of security and safety. It's a trap. I was stuck in that trap for the majority of my life. I could've chosen to remain in that headspace of being miserable, to be physical pain itself, to hold grudges against those who've wronged me, to allow my frustrations and anger to lead me into each interaction for the rest of my life, to take out those frustrations on everything and everyone—but at the end of the day, I had a choice. Don't get me wrong, I'm still very much human and I slip up on many occasions. It's all a part of the experience and a never-ending process, but eventually, I had to wake myself up. Depending on how strong your ambitions are, it's more than possible to pull yourself out of that endless and destructive cycle that you've been stuck in. You just have to be honest with yourself, put your ego and stubbornness aside, and be willing to choose differently while also being open to different perspectives.

The healing of your body and mind starts with having the willingness to change. You're the only one who can create real, lasting change in your own life. You can have the best support system, but at some point, you'll notice that changes cannot take place unless you yourself choose to change. No matter how deep your hole seems, if you want to see any improvement, you're going to need to pick yourself up and start the process of getting out of that hole eventually. You 100% will fail on numerous occasions, but effort itself is still progression. The more you put in the effort, the more desired outcomes you'll achieve. When you overcome difficult situations or unhealthy habits, the more resilience you build inside yourself. Good health, true internal peace, a loving and calm nature, are all attainable if you really want them –

for all of us.

This part of the book might be "aggressive" for some, but the truth just *is* sometimes, and it's come through with the best intentions. If you've been through any type of hardship in your life, you've most likely looked back and thought about ways you could've changed certain things. What has happened, happened. So, loosen the noose just a little bit and start to forgive yourself for being a version of you that you never intended to be. Your situation was most likely led by unconscious wounded parts of you that run on autopilot. In that moment, you were doing the best you could. But a goal to work towards in your life is to not allow yourself to be in autopilot mode, and instead strive to be conscious at each and every moment. That means slowing down—and before you're like, "whoa, wait a minute, that's just how I am, I can't slow down, I have to do this and that, I need to achieve X, Y, Z and I have to get this done or else I won't survive," (or my father-in-law's favorite line, "the bills won't pay themselves")—really sit with why you're making excuses. Absolutely nothing is more important than your own well-being. And if that means having to take a step back from all your doings to slow down and consciously choose your next thought, action, or words—you'd be wise to follow through.

Every person has their story, and every story deserves to

be heard. The lessons we learn from the battles we face deserve to be shared because odds are they'll help at least one person outside of yourself. I've carefully selected the topics I talk about, taking into consideration that these lessons will, without a doubt, make a positive impact on your life. It's up to you to read between the lines to decipher what other areas you can explore or improve to unlock a life of endless possibilities. Please read the following pages objectively, with an open mind and an open heart. My energy isn't for everyone, and I don't take offense to that. So keep in mind the following, as much as your ego permits.

1

FACING THE BRUTAL TRUTH

My flight was booked for three weeks after Tyler left at the end of my flare. I felt forced to be without him. He went on to start the process of pursuing our goal of planting roots in Hawaii. What felt like the longest three and a half weeks of my entire life was filled with the crumbs of total defeat. I felt broken and lost, as though I had just finished sprinting a six-month-long marathon. My parents both worked full-time jobs, and my sisters were off living their own lives, so I was left completely alone. I was physically alone and spiritually isolated—three weeks of solitude in which I had to face myself and my emotions. I wrote a lot during this time, and when I wasn't writing, I filled my time with solo trips to the beach and to the gym multiple times a day, which usually ended with me crying myself to sleep. I barely heard from Tyler, and when we did communicate, it was short and empty.

I set myself the goal of gaining a certain amount of weight back by the time my flight was scheduled to depart for Hawaii, and that was the only thing I focused on. I was still on seizure medication, and at night, when I'd go to bed, I'd take my dose, which made me feel couch-locked and confused. I'd sit and listen to Yaima albums until my internal pain lulled me to sleep. It was the most uncomfortable feeling of emptiness, loneliness, and deep sadness. I battled back and forth with myself, what seemed like every night, about whether I should just call it quits. I barely talked to anyone, even my own parents. I'd find myself going to the gym for a second or third time that day, just as they were getting home from work. Then, I'd come home, shower, and go right to bed. I did everything I could to avoid everyone. I was humiliated and ashamed of what I had allowed to transpire and was intimidated of this foreign life I had come back to. I also still couldn't make logical sense of things I had seen, so I hid inside myself, away from everyone.

By the beginning of that third week in New Jersey, I felt more than ready to present this latest version of myself I had curated out of my solitude. I chose to embrace the path of unknown territory instead of letting it consume me, but to be fully transparent, that did not come easily. When I had arrived in Hawaii and reunited with my husband, the harsh reality had really set in. This wasn't the same person I knew prior to this flare, and I'm sure for him I was not the same person either. We both had a challenging time accepting this fact which eventually led to us growing even further apart. We quickly became what felt like roommates as I drowned myself in marijuana around the clock, always covering up the uncomfortable foreign feelings I was experiencing when we were around each other. Abusing a substance is obviously never smart, especially freshly coming out of psychosis. I started to question my reality again, seeing and hearing the beings who used to taunt me were back in full swing and only got more intense. I felt like I was losing myself yet again. The "new and clear" version of myself I had brought to Hawaii with me seemed to be slipping away. I started to realize these symptoms weren't only present in a medication induced psychosis anymore, they were a part of my new reality. But even through all the covering up, I still managed to let my new perception seep through in small ways and did my best to be the example of change I wanted for us. Tyler slowly saw that. Eventually, after many long, deep, heart-wrenching conversations, we once again chose to work through this together. Although we knew the road ahead would be long and uncomfortable, we dedicated our few years in Hawaii to falling in love again.

2

WHAT IF?

After endless reflection on my flare, I started to come to the realization that I would never have thought possible before the experience. What if I did die? What if I never went back in my body after my first seizure? What if that's just how my mind was attempting to make sense of my reality so that I didn't have too much of a shock to my system? What if instead, I actually entered a new reality? No one really knows what happens when you die, but what if this is what happens? Entering a new reality that's sort of the same as the previous but with so many stark differences that I was forced to believe it must be a different place (Some refer to this as quantum immortality.)

Right after the first seizure, my cognizant memory had me believing that I went back into my same body, in the same life I had been living. But the memory lapses from when the ambulance came, the entire hospital stay, and most of what transpired during psychosis had left me feeling that this went way deeper than my logical mind. I've come to realize the reason why my experience with psychosis was so intense and demonic was because that was my version of Hell, my own version of purgatory. A place where all of my fears were manifested from, a place where I experienced the worst possible outcomes with those who were around me. I interacted with the worst version of Tyler that my mind could create, the worst version of my mother, father, sister, friends, and even my dog. I was taunted and followed and so paranoid that I could have ended my life for the sake of my sanity, had my hallucinations not tricked me out of it. If I had stayed in such a low state without at least a glimpse of awareness—that "this couldn't possibly be it"—I would've spent the rest of my life in eternal Hell. But because I had a deep knowing that this couldn't be the life I had left behind, it allowed me to work my way out of that and into the reality I was meant to cross over into. I was trapped in such mental anguish. Had it been all physical, that would've eventually led to a physical death, a complete shutdown of the body's systems. But with mental pain, you remain in that state of suffering until you do something about it. That is what, I believe, Hell actually is: it's not the same physical place that's most talked about today; it's simply a state of complete and total resistance.

When I had finally stopped resisting, I was able to feel into my new surroundings. I was in a new life and lucky enough to still possess what seemed like the same body and somewhat the same identity. There was no denying this: this was proof that my time being Hailey wasn't done yet and there was still growth to be had. Because I had reached such a low on the spectrum of emotion, I unlocked new perceptions and knowledge to assist me in continuing to grow for the remainder of my time on earth—even if this meant being in an entirely different reality. The parallel processing of my old reality and this new reality was difficult to navigate in the beginning, causing bouts of depression and overall feelings of thinking I was legitimately crazy. To be honest, some days I still do feel crazy. But instead of being upset at that feeling now, I embrace it. Let's face it: we're all a little bit crazy. I've realized that there are a lot of people walking around this world playing out their own internal Hell, and most don't even realize it.

3

ANGER FUELS OUR DISCONTENT

Over time, Tyler and I started opening up to each other more. It eventually came to the surface that he was holding so much anger towards me—for almost dying a couple of months after our wedding, the culmination of pain from the flare-ups in 2019 and 2021, and unknowingly using him as an emotional punching bag when I wasn't in my right mind. It's no wonder he completely checked out of our relationship when he left for Hawaii; it was his way of processing. It was not until the anger was allowed to be expressed that we were able to start working on rebuilding. It is always one step forward, two steps back.

I have personally held onto a lot of pent-up anger from many different phases of my life over the years. It has taken a lot of discipline to tone it down, but with time and a desire to change, I've been able to have better control over my anger. Although, that part of me will always exist, which is why during that flare in 2021, it exploded out of me like an atomic bomb. Seriously, I could not mean that in more of a literal sense.

Circumstances growing up led me to be incredibly angry at everything. The rage from my early childhood that I had locked away deep inside myself was a huge contributor to the state of my health at that time. That anger has followed me into adulthood, which is why I believe that holding all of that in for over 20 years really did play a huge part in manifesting sickness and an imbalance within my body. I did not just wake up sick one day; it was the cumulative anger, stress, and sadness that I buried, manifesting into physical ailments when my body physically could not hold any more. It is honestly very embarrassing to admit that anger has had a chokehold on me for most of my life. My short fuse and temper will always be a work in progress, but it's much easier for me to have a handle on now. That ease would not have been possible without my aggressive explosion, which forced me to face that reality. Your internal world will always show through your external awareness. It takes a lot of energy to push those feelings down, so if you can identify with your anger, even a little bit, notice the ways it impacts your life. Otherwise, your body will eventually give up trying to fight back, and it will manifest it into some type of imbalance that will lead you down a road of sickness.

Anger, frustration, and being miserable really do not look good on anyone. Aside from our own personal struggles, we have gone through quite a bit as a society lately, which has resulted in all of us being so divided, resentful, entitled, and just flat out mean to each other. We are all so used to tightly grasping on to our dramas and the feelings that come along with them. We have all forgotten that we're looking at life through different lenses. We're overwhelmed by everything—stressed about not being able to pay our bills or worried that we can't put dinner on the table. Most people are working multiple jobs and still not making ends meet. That anger *is* justifiable, but there will still be consequences for holding yourself to that level of energy. Only *you* have the power to help yourself—and in turn, the power to help all of us. If you are angry, depressed, or grieving, find an outlet: physical movement, making music, consistent meditation, bodywork, energy work, silent retreats, writing, or some type of new hobby where you can express yourself without judgment. There are so many avenues available to you. You do not have to be a miserable sack for the rest of your life. Choose to want to feel better, strive to feel happy, and go from there. But you need to be honest with yourself and not feel guilty for being unhappy in the first place— address it instead. Just because the universe orchestrated my experience for me to release all my anger, sadness, grief, and fear that I was holding in the way that it did, doesn't mean you need to go through something equally traumatizing or intense to release your own. Maybe if I was aware of this concept prior to my last flare, things wouldn't have escalated so quickly. Once you can address your anger and somewhat pinpoint where it stems from, your perspective on everything will change. And this will eventually lead you to living with purpose. You'll be kinder, more loving, and more compassionate—to yourself first, and then to others. Picture anger as a giant cloud. That cloud will be dark and rainy, blocking out all the positive things in your life. Take away the cloud—the deep anger you've buried—and there's no rain, leaving an infinite number of sunny days and space for more positive experiences to present themselves to you. The possibilities are truly limitless, but it all starts with you and your willingness to make a change in the first place.

4

WEAVING CLARITY FROM CHAOS

During my flare, I wasn't in control of absolutely anything in my mind or body. The more I attempted to be, the deeper I fell into psychosis, causing me to become further disconnected from the true reality I was used to. There are times when you might not be able to make cognitive choices for whatever reason, and that's okay too— as long as you eventually snap out of it and take your power back. I have been in numerous situations in my life where I was in different states of mind, at varying degrees of severity, where I had to snap out of it, or my life would have ended. Each time that I was faced with such drastic measures, some divine nature seemed to make itself known, changing the course of my life.

The power of free will is, what I believe, the most important aspect of life to further understand and learn to work with. Sure, you can do the absolute bare minimum and allow things to happen as they will with no interference on your part, but that will eventually translate to a bypassing laziness. You have been given the gift of being a human— use it. I do believe there are set paths for each of us as individuals to walk down, but depending on your moment-to-moment choices regarding your thoughts, actions, and reactions—your free will—you have the ability to course-correct yourself onto those set paths with the least resistance or the best outcomes in your favor. If you are always making choices to please others rather than choosing what makes you happy or fulfilled, you are technically choosing to walk the more difficult path. Yet, if you choose your happiness over everything and put yourself and your dreams first, you are choosing to walk on the path with the highest potential outcomes for you. Although you may choose that higher path, it does not protect you from negative experiences. (I use the terms positive and negative loosely because they are ultimately subjective.) Instead, as long as you vow to always choose what's right in your heart, follow your intuition in your moment-to-moment choices, and take an extra minute to think about how you can respond, the hardships that will inevitably present themselves will be "easier" to navigate, if that makes sense.

As a living example, during the birth of my daughter, there was a moment of anxiety because I had a slightly higher temperature than normal. I was stuck at 7 cm dilated and had already been in labor for 31 hours. This fever immediately brought back all the emotions from my fever-led flare and the memories that came along with them. I knew at this moment that I needed to keep my composure—not only for the sake of my own health, but for the health of my baby who was still inside of me. Tyler was overwhelmed by the emotions and memories that surfaced and really had a tough time dealing with them in such a chaotic moment. I composed myself and my energy and told him to take a break and to try to get some sleep. I laid down and meditated for about an hour while he napped, focusing on my breath and the knowing that I was soon going to be meeting my healthy baby. When I felt my intuition nudge me, I told my doula to get the doctor to check if I was fully dilated. When they checked, I was 10 cm and ready to push. If I had not taken the time to gather and tune into myself, and instead allowed the anxiety to take over and cause physiological changes to my body, I would not have had such an amazing birth following that situation. I've shared some of our birth story on a podcast called *"Inside the Tide,"* so I won't go into that now, but for the sake of this example, what better illustration of manipulating my own energy in real time?

Because we are human and all learning as we go, we often get caught up in the noise of life—the job, the bills, the dramas. We allow these stressors to dictate our thoughts and our actions, which inevitably leads to unhappiness. If we remove the "thing" from the equation, we are left with the *self* and the *awareness of self.* Have you ever allowed the awareness of self to take charge of the thoughts you allow to swirl around your mind? Have you ever paid attention to how you talk to yourself or witness your idling thoughts? If you have never given this any attention, I challenge you to stop being a victim to your mind and give it a shot.

For example, when you are sitting with a group of people and everyone is gossiping about a specific person, are your idling thoughts judging, going along with, or just observing what's going on in the conversation? What about when you look in the mirror—are your thoughts making judgements against yourself, are they expressing gratitude for how far you have come, or are you just observing what you see? How about when you are driving in your car on your way home from work—are you thinking about how you are going to afford your bills for the month, stressing about what you are going to make for dinner, or are you just enjoying the drive?

Our minds *will* run rampant 24/7 if we do not interject. And if you have gone most of your life without interjecting, aren't you exhausted yet? Having the discipline to say to yourself, "Wait a minute, why am I thinking about this?" and then redirecting your thoughts to something more positive will not only help in that moment, but the more you practice this, the more automatic it will become. This is definitely something that takes time, but with enough attention and self-accountability, eventually you will have fewer random thoughts and more consciously directed ones.

View yourself as a magnet. Negative thoughts will bring that same negativity to you in some form. But by course-correcting your own thoughts and consciously choosing a more positive thought or emotion toward something, you will inevitably attract that same positive energy back to you. When I gave the example earlier about when I was in labor, I could have taken that situation and made it completely negative and not in my favor. If I had given in to the negativity that was going on around me and allowed my thoughts to sound like "Holy shit, I'm having a fever, what if something happens to the baby, what if this starts a flare, what if I can't do this"—that would've caused the worst possible outcome. But because I was able to zoom out and observe what was going on, I was able to consciously choose to have better thoughts and not fall for the trap: "I can do this, I just need to relax, everything will be okay, it's all working out, best-case scenario, I am healthy, my baby is safe." See the difference?

Another example, if someone you know is always having good things happen to them, and you notice yourself become bitter or jealous, can you recognize how this is a negative reaction? Can you guess what kind of situations this could possibly attract, or fail to attract, if you were to choose to think this way? Instead of feeling negative emotions, you could try embodying being genuinely happy for them. By doing this, you immediately just flipped the script, and more positive outcomes are already on their way to you. Without sounding redundant, the point is to always take a minute to zoom out and give yourself the chance to choose your next thought, action, or reaction. If you are in a position where you are sick or if you are going through a rough time, try zooming out and recognizing the ways you can shift your thoughts and attitude in the smallest of moments. Once I stopped complaining, judging, and being so sour, I saw significant improvement in my life and my health. Take it one thought at a time—huge changes definitely won't happen overnight. Remember this: **Thoughts are the frequency that you are experiencing, so choose wisely.**

5

TRANSFORMING PAIN INTO POWER

You might notice that once you get the hang of becoming more aware of your thoughts, you make better decisions. When you make better decisions, it dominoes into you becoming a more enjoyable person to be around. When you become more enjoyable to be around, you make a positive impact in other people's lives. And if you make a positive impact on someone's life, that person is more inclined to do the same for someone else. It's all a chain reaction that started with the simple fact of you being more aware of what's going on in your head. So simple, yet so complex.

I have not always been the best version of myself. As I mentioned earlier, a large chunk of my life before I hit my twenties was spent being miserable, negative, and just an overall bitch (for lack of a better word). I admit that I have been mean and rude to many people throughout my life. If you are one of them, I sincerely apologize. Not only was I operating from an unconscious part of myself, but I was also operating from a place of such hurt that I had no idea how to address. Between my childhood experiences, my home life as a teenager, bad friends, stressors, and responsibilities at certain times—I could rack up a whole list of great excuses, but it is never okay to take that hurt out on others. The person I am today would never intend to purposely hurt someone else. The person I used to be, maybe, but not this Hailey. Oftentimes, we hold onto things that have hurt us so deeply for so long that, eventually, they unconsciously leak out of us as negativity. They become a part of our personality if we fail to take accountability for the hurt that we have bestowed.

More times than not, I have personally been trapped in a place where I have felt so insignificant, worthless, not good enough, and lonely. At times, life seemed too emotionally painful. It does not matter who you are or how severe the mistakes you've made are—no one deserves to feel like that. Even the worst of the worst deserves compassion in some form, because on the other side of their wrongdoings is a person who is hurting for whatever reason. If we all looked at each other with a little more compassion, this world would not be so cruel. Having compassion for yourself is equally as important as having compassion for others. You are always doing the best you know how to in that moment, and luckily, there is always something to be learned. So again, do not be so hard on yourself. Instead, attempt to make slight changes to be a better version of yourself, even with all the pain you may carry.

With all of that being said, forgiveness is your key to every door of opportunity that's closed off. Self-forgiveness and forgiveness of others can truly transform your life in ways you probably thought impossible. If I never forgave my parents for how they made me feel and for the things I had to experience and witness in my childhood, I'd still be bitter, I'd still be lashing out, and we'd still have a terrible relationship. If I never forgave myself for how I have treated others during my younger years, I'd still be a miserable, bitter, entitled bitch. Forgiveness has almost nothing to do with the other person. Think about that for a moment. Other than truly forgiving someone from the heart—meaning there are no ill thoughts about them floating around your mind, there's no animosity if you happen to cross paths again, and there's no pit in your stomach when you think of them—the only thing you have to do is be at peace with what is and how things have played out. Simply be aware and take accountability for the part you played in the situation, sit with that, and see what you can do differently next time. Also, attempt to be aware of the other side of the story; most people don't intentionally hurt you—they're just injured themselves. If you're stubborn like me, that may feel like one of the most difficult things you could do. But once you put aside your stubbornness, can see the situation for what it is, and actually accept it for what it is, you can allow yourself to forgive. Once you do that, you'll feel how heavy that grudge had been weighing on you. Holding grudges inevitably leads to illness in some way. First, it will function as a roadblock to opportunities of "would-have-beens." The longer and tighter you grasp onto that grudge, the more it turns into sickness within yourself. You're doing the biggest disservice to your health and your happiness. Regardless of how painful it once was, let it all go and choose to use that pain as fuel to become a better version of yourself.

Letting go of grudges and forgiving someone does not mean that you are obligated to let those people back into your life or make physical amends. As I just mentioned above, it simply means that you have come to peace with what is, and you have let things be as they are. Feel the feelings, then move on. All is always happening for a reason, and I truly stick to this motto (so much so that I have it tattooed on my body). If something or someone exits your life in some way, for whatever reason, there's a divinely guided reason for it. That exit opens up space for new opportunities to present themselves to you.

To recap: zoom out and be disciplined in your thoughts; be a good person; have compassion for yourself and others; forgive yourself and others; and let things be as they are. I can guarantee you that if you apply these five things to your daily life, you'll start to see very drastic changes in all areas of your life and your relationships.

6

MORE ON FORGIVENESS

Growing up in the environment that I did, I didn't have the best relationship with my parents for a really long time. Physical and verbal abuse were very prominent in my childhood. I've witnessed many terrible fights, have been directly in the middle of them, and felt I was given way too much responsibility at an incredibly young age. There were many hardships we faced together as a family. I used to resent both of my parents for different reasons, and it wasn't until my first diagnosis in 2015 that I had a reality check. Again, forgiveness can transform your life in ways you couldn't possibly imagine, and I'm a living example. The moment I truly forgave my mom and dad and realized they were doing the best they could with what they knew and had at the time, my life truly shifted. That's not to say what I experienced didn't have a negative impact on me, but because I allowed my life to shift in that way and didn't cloud it with hatred or hold a grudge against them, it had a domino effect. I noticed their lives shifted too, as well as their relationships with their own parents. My parents and I are now very close, and it's all been an incredible thing to see unfold.

Although it took me falling ill to realize this, I encourage you not to sit around waiting for something to happen. Get ahead of the game and dig deep inside yourself to find the love and compassion needed to forgive others and yourself. If you're holding on to trivial bullshit, the clock is ticking for you, truly. Keep in mind that you can't change anyone else but yourself. In many ways, most would view that as frustrating, but really, it's a blessing. We get to release the burden of trying to change someone else and only have to focus on maintaining ourselves. How amazing is that? Hop off the wheel of repetition and take a step toward the change you're dying to see. Your future self will most definitely thank you.

***

Romantic relationships are a whole new level of difficult, and I say that from a place of love. I have been lucky enough to cross paths with Tyler, my husband and best friend—a child I grew into adulthood with and a man completely unmatched, no doubt. We started our relationship at just 15 and 16 years old, not knowing it would blossom into such a beautiful pairing. Like any other young teen relationship, we went through our tests. We walked each other through so many years of egoic tendencies, and energetically, we beat the hell out of each other. Year after year we shed aspects of ourselves that didn't fit into who we were envisioning becoming. It was definitely not easy and took true dedication to self and to the other. Deconstructing societal norms and choosing to walk a path all our own is the road less traveled nowadays. So many people have asked how we've stayed together for so long and still don't hate each other, or how we've stayed together during our personal mistakes or the hardships with my health. The best answer I can give is that we consciously choose each other and our relationship, and we work on it—it's as simple as that. If one of us were to stop putting in the effort to better our relationship, the relationship would fail. It's a joint effort all around.

Ironically, what brought us closer together was the same thing that tore us apart: the trials with my health. You always hear stories of young relationships ending because one of them falls ill, but in my case, Tyler chose to help me walk down that road instead of easily running away. This came with its own set of challenges, and we've worked our asses off to repair our relationship, and we continue to prioritize that now. Maintaining and bettering a relationship is demanding work, and many people give up when things become tricky or uncomfortable, or they let their emotions get the best of them and end up leaving. If you genuinely love someone, you'll figure out how to make it work together regardless of what's trying to pull you apart. Love is multifaceted; it's not always sweet and flawless. While there will undoubtedly be moments of joy and pleasure, pain is also an essential part of what makes love, love. This complexity is what gives love its depth and meaning. Embracing both the highs and lows is crucial when committing to love another person, because without this understanding, love would lose much of its significance.

Playing the part of "the sick one" has been challenging but imagine being the counterpart to that. Having to watch the person you love most go through so much pain and uncertainty for years on end, and not being able to take the struggle away from them. Feeling helpless and defeated, taking the brunt of it all—that's true pain. (If you're in that position for your spouse or loved one, please know you are extremely appreciated.) There have been periods of time when we've held our hardships and shortcomings against each other, which only led to arguments and hostility. Although needing to be expressed, once we worked through it together, expressed forgiveness, and continued to vow to be better for each other, healing had space to take place.

7

THE WORK YOU'RE AVOIDING

I'm truly fortunate to have had the experiences I've had at such an early age. These experiences have revealed to me the fragility of life—how, in the blink of an eye, everything can change, and you may find yourself gone from this reality, leaving behind the trivial obsessions that once seemed so important. What matters most to me is my own happiness. For the first time in my life, I'm more than content with who I am as a person—I know few people can say that. To be honest, I'm surprised I'm even saying that because, for whatever reason, I hold myself to such ambitious standards. But I wouldn't be looking through this lens if I had not been dragged like a rag doll through the pits of Hell at my absolute lowest. And, of course, I have a lengthy list of things I want to change and improve within myself, as I'm constantly working on them, but overall, I'm so happy to be me—and so grateful to be conscious of this version of myself.

If you want to love and live in the light, you have to face and sit in the darkest parts of yourself first. Facing your darkest demons and your most uncomfortable emotions is truly the only way to evolve. If that doesn't interest you, of course you have free will to make that decision, although you'll be spinning on the same wheel for quite a while if that's what you choose. I believe I came to this earth to continue my journey of bettering my truest self, and that's what I have set out to do for the rest of my life. We live in incredible times right now regarding mass spiritual awakening—and yes, I understand those words are heavily loaded. Through all the self-care, self-help books, gatherings, and online communities, the real work has become lost in translation. "Love and light," "positivity," and "psychedelics" are wonderful, but if you can't really face, head-on, the darkest parts of yourself, and then go on to integrate what you've learned, you're going to be running in circles until the end of time. I ask that for every person reading this book, take the time to do your deep inner work. The future of humanity depends on you. It depends on all of us. Everything is connected, and if you've been called to read this book, you most likely already knew that because you're looking for something more. The more we individually uncover our deepest truths that are hiding underneath our wrongdoings, our judgments, our egos, and our failures, the more we raise the energetic state of the collective, which will result in an ever-evolving unity consciousness. Do the work. The dirty work. It will be uncomfortable, devastating and at times, very painful—but worth it in every sense. The most unimaginable beauty, emotions, and levels of love await you. You'll be awestruck at the ways life can and will reward you for going a little deeper.

I am in no way advertising dumping super positive affirmations and actions onto yourself. Toxic positivity is dangerous, which is why I personally strayed far away from the "love and light" culture that's prominent today. I've had my fair share of that misconstrued lifestyle in the past, and it was not helpful for my growth. Forcing yourself to completely ignore the negatives in your life and filling them with talk-positive bullshit is only going to make your journey a lot messier. Facing your baggage head-on, sitting with all of the discomfort, the painful emotions, the physical pain, and acknowledging your shortcomings—sounds daunting. But wouldn't you rather deal with your problems instead of letting them get buried deep inside you? Your body holds these memories in its cells. In most cases, aside from karmic lessons you came into this world with, the chronic illnesses we see today are nothing more than the things you refuse to let go of. That may be a hard pill to swallow because it's putting you in the spotlight, but trust me when I say that if you truly start letting go, transformation will happen almost instantly. Your pain, whether physical or mental, is the body's way of saying, "If you want to choose to ignore X, Y, Z, I'm going to make sure you literally can't ignore it anymore." And then you'll sit in that pain for as long as you continue to be stubborn about facing your battles. For as long as you hold those grudges, for as long as you refuse to operate from a different thought pattern, you will be a slave to your struggles.

It's important not to forget to have fun in the process of the self-work you undertake. Take each step forwards and backwards as a blessing. Becoming too serious is also dangerous and can lead you down a self-destructive cycle. Try not allowing yourself to get too wrapped up in the doings or the details. You'll come across many points in your life where you thought you had it all figured out, you thought you overcame this or that, you thought you were the best version of yourself, but truly it's a never-ending process of progression that ebbs and flows the harder you don't try. If you find yourself in an "almighty" state, consider it a sign that your next lesson is on the horizon.

No matter what you believe in, regarding religion or spirituality, you are an infinite being of energy that's ever-evolving in this vast section of space that we all find ourselves in. Our energetic imprint in this physical world means so much more than any of us could ever comprehend. Each and every one of us—regardless of demographics, upbringing, or current state of being—is so extremely important to the evolution of not only humanity, but to the totality of consciousness itself. So, even if you don't feel like it at this moment, you are indeed loved, important, and very much needed here. Your entire existence is a miracle; there's no arguing that fact. I believe we came into this life knowing everything we'd be getting ourselves into. But when we get here in physical form, we purposely forget the game plan. It wouldn't be a test if you knew all the answers. Everything you experience in a single lifetime is a miracle. Whether the experience is perceived as bad or amazing, it's for a reason. We're on this path of self-growth as individual souls. The more we align ourselves with our own path, the easier it becomes to recognize the subtle signs guiding us toward our next steps. We are always being guided by something much larger than any of us. Whether you believe in God or some other higher power, the life force energy that creates us all, that flows through our lungs when we take a deep breath, that surrounds us at our lowest points—is always there. You are never truly alone. Be honest with yourself, look at yourself in the heart, and win the war against yourself. Only *you* can be the hero of your story.

8

THE ART OF BEING YOURSELF

I believe that our detours from paths of growth often stem from the overwhelming influence of the world around us. No matter what direction we look in, we're fed unattainable standards. Whether it's what we should look like, how we should behave, what we should think, or "who" we should be—we're constantly made to feel like we aren't good enough. Those feelings eventually pressure us into aspiring to be these false, made-up versions of ourselves, keeping us in a constant state of comparison. And before we know it, we're just another cog in the wheel, another "sheep in the herd," if you will. When we fall victim to this intense pressure, we end up sacrificing our individuality. Our individuality is what defines our humanity, so when it's stripped away, we risk becoming trapped in a sea of identical facades. We get caught in this vicious cycle of "not being good enough," we get dumbed down, and we lose the spark we came here with. We become unhappy, depressed, confused. Considering the alarming decline in global mental health over the past few years—clearly, something is wrong.

You *can* break free. You *can* choose not to play this game. Instead of trying to fit in, have you ever considered being your true self? The complete version of you—the one who makes silly faces in the mirror and recites random lines from childhood cartoons. The person who pretends to be on a talk show, answering questions while wandering through the house, making absurd expressions, and then seamlessly continues with the day as if none of these ever happened. I know I can't be the only one. I'm weird and I say and do weird things. And I know most of you do too, and if you don't... well, congratulations, I guess. We are all born unique, yet somehow, it's been normalized for everyone to be anything but themselves. These standards of being "normal" and having to look and act in a certain way have clouded all of our perceptions of ourselves. So many people strive to be copies of influencers or celebrities, when in reality, it's all a show. Social media and television aren't realistic. Most celebrities aren't even real (but I'm not going down that rabbit hole in this book). Sit with yourself for a moment and ask what it is you really want; what you see yourself as, the type of person you strive to be, or where you want to be in a year from now. In a world overflowing with replicas, strive to be someone who cannot be duplicated.

Let your personality flourish. I've struggled with this deeply, as my hardships have profoundly shaped my self-perception. I've experienced a wide range of physical changes—losing my hair repeatedly, fluctuating weight, struggling with the effects of steroids on my voice, dealing with acne and scars from procedures, and battling with the side effects of lupus, which robbed me of collagen in my face at an early age. On top of that, I've battled memory loss that has made holding conversations challenging. My self-esteem was at an all-time low when I came out of that last flare, and I'd be lying if I said I never wished to be someone else. I was so scared to be myself because I didn't even know who I was. All I knew was that I was alive, and that knowing allowed me to switch my perception and be grateful for that train wreck of a phase. It derailed me from the trap of conforming to the norm and gifted me the opportunity to start fresh. I had to rediscover who I was and learn to exist again, even if it meant becoming a person vastly different from who I had been before.

There was a time in my life when I didn't think twice about how others perceived me, which explains some of my regrettable fad phases. Then, I came out of my flare at just about one hundred pounds with a half head of hair, terrible skin, and not an ounce of muscle on my body. I had to face the reality that I wasn't the beautiful, athletic, somewhat confident, 20-something-year-old I thought I had been. I was humbled fairly quickly. But I had to own that version of me the best I could, and that's where the switch in my perception started. I had the choice of being distraught at how I looked and could've taken that anger and frustration out on everyone. But instead, I chose to embrace the fact that I looked like a teenage boy with a botched haircut who looked like they were recovering from some type of heavy drug addiction. I was looking really rough, but I was alive. Like I said, I owned it, and I did my best to work my way back up to looking and feeling healthy and confident again. I kept myself accountable and stuck to zoning in on this new mindset and perception I had. I worked really hard at being me in all situations and realized that it's important to embrace who we are rather than try to fit into the crowd. I learned that I was somewhat awkward, that I didn't really know many things to hold a conversation anymore, and that I didn't care for meaningless conversation. I felt so much freer when I stopped thinking I was wrong for being this way. You'll feel so much freer when you let go of the expectations that others have of you. Learn to love all parts of yourself and do what you can to be your own best friend. If you can achieve that, you won't be strangled by the need for any outside validation anymore—which is a destructive path all on its own.

If you find yourself surrounded by people who seem to

block you from being yourself or people who you feel the need to be a certain way around, maybe rethink who you're allowing into your life. Most of us have gone through life with many masks on, always altering our personalities or interests to fit in with the people around us. Not everyone needs to like you, and you don't need to like everyone. (Maybe read that line one more time.) When you can let go of the need to be liked and stop trying to be everyone's best friend, your life will shift dramatically. You'll notice how many people you thought were your friends will drop like flies because you aren't trying to please them anymore. You'll feel a massive load off your shoulders because you're not having to uphold some rehearsed facade. Live for yourself, take the mask off permanently, and the rest will follow.

9

BOLDLY UNBOTHERED

The main reason we wear these masks in the first place is because we fear being rejected if we let our true selves shine. My question to you is: why worry about rejection? Why surround yourself with people who don't accept you for who you are or who judge you for being your authentic self? It may be harder for some of you but try to stop caring what others think of you altogether. People are only going to be able to meet you where they are. This isn't a matter of who is better or worse or who's further along in their journey; it's simply a matter of accepting that we are all at different stages. Everything is always happening in its own time, and it may not be your time to be at a certain stage that someone else is at—and vice versa. You're most likely going to be misunderstood at some point in your life, and you're going to have to accept that. I've been misunderstood for the majority of my life and although frustrating at first, I've learned to embrace it. I've come to realize that lessons happen at a rapid-fire pace in my life, which results in constant growth. I outgrow a lot of people and places because of this. And again, not to say I'm better than any of you, I have just accepted that I'm growing, and I allow it to unfold as it is. Part of growth is not being attached to people, places, or things and letting go of what no longer energetically matches you.

I get the occasional social anxiety. I am self-conscious. I make mistakes, I get things messed up and I sound stupid (lots of the time). The only time I seem to ever make a little bit of sense is when I write. I'm human, and so are you. You're allowed to mess up, you're allowed to be human. No one is perfect, and the idea of perfection isn't what it seems. The universe is perfect, not because it adheres to specific guidelines or standards, but because it exists, in all of its confusion and brilliance. In all of your quirkiness and uniqueness, you exist. So, why waste your time worrying about what others think of you? Everyone is dealing with their own shit. The things you're worried about others noticing about you most likely aren't being noticed because people are too busy worrying about their own insecurities. Got a few pimples? Gained a few extra pounds over the holiday? Accidentally let one loose when you were getting up from your chair? Drank too much at your sister's wedding and embarrassed yourself? Forgot to put a bra on when you left the house? Put two completely different shoes on when you left for work? **Who cares?** Seriously, who cares? Odds are you aren't the only one that any of these "embarrassing" things happen to. We are all learning as we go and experiencing this weird world together. Ease up and stop taking this life so seriously. In other words, it's time for that stick to come out of your ass.

10

WHISPERS OF THE HEART

Once you stop caring about what others think of you, you'll notice you can hear yourself a lot more clearly. If you can't, don't panic—sometimes there's a transition period of absolutely nothing flowing in that noggin (this may be where I currently am right now). When you eventually come out of that weird phase, your mind won't be flooded with anxiety anymore, and you'll be able to tap into making decisions based on the feelings you feel inside yourself rather than be influenced by those around you. When you learn to start listening to your intuition, navigating through life becomes so much easier. Then, when you start fully trusting your intuition, your life becomes more enjoyable. It's usually extremely subtle, but the more you quiet your mind and the more you make a practice out of sitting with yourself, the stronger your intuition will become. I'm at a point in my life where I will listen to my intuition over absolutely anything because I have full trust that it's guiding me in the direction I'm supposed to be going. I trust things are always working out so much that a lot of the people in my life think I'm batshit crazy. Eventually, they see that whatever it is I'm trusting in, *always* works out. So, in the end it's a win-win for me: Everyone leaves me alone for fear of catching my crazy and I also get rewarded with this beautiful life I'm currently living.

Back when my flare had calmed down and Tyler had left for Hawaii, I stayed back in New Jersey for a few weeks to be extra cautious ensuring I was in the clear to be that far away from my doctors (this wasn't my decision). I had the strongest intuitive feeling inside that I needed to go with him instead of staying back. But because of the last few months leading up to that, no one thought it was a good idea that I leave just yet. But I felt the opposite; I felt I needed to get out of there as fast as I could so I could start to process, away from everyone involved, what we just went through. I felt left behind, and I felt like no one could hear me. I've always been one to listen to my gut instinct, and it's exceedingly rare for me to ignore such an intense feeling. And, of course, that ultimate decision of being forced to ignore my intuition to let him go without me—backfired. The consequences of one decision like that ended up having the largest impact on our relationship, which we've since worked hard to repair. The point I'm trying to make is that listening to your intuition is **the** most important thing you can do for yourself, even if it seems crazy to people around you. And in times that you ignore it, like I did, you'll have to face the consequences and clean up the mess that follows.

If you're able to stay present within your decisions that you're gifted with, you'll realize how many of those decisions are based on what's in your heart rather than the thoughts in your head. If something really doesn't feel right inside or you notice circumstances seeming like they're constantly against you rather than for you, listen to those signs. In some situations, you might feel that although there seems to be a lot going wrong, you still feel strongly about your decision—these could also be tests to see if you'll stay true to that original gut feeling. Use your discernment and listen to that feeling. It requires significant trial and error, along with a commitment to self-discovery, to truly recognize the signs that appear for you and to understand your body's energetic responses to the external world. The number of times we've uprooted our family because our living situation no longer felt right often made us feel like we were losing our minds. Yet, each time we trusted those gut feelings, we were rewarded with even better circumstances.

If you feel that a change is needed in your life and you're dissatisfied with your current situation, pay attention to that feeling. While it's important to balance logic with your creative instincts to make the best decisions for yourself, don't hesitate to take the leap toward what you genuinely want. I would never discourage you from quitting your job and moving across the world; we've done it multiple times, and each time it has turned out well for us. We have the foundational mindset of wholeheartedly believing that everything is always working out best-case scenario as long as we are listening to our hearts and not our heads. So, if you can get yourself to a place of fully trusting yourself and what's in store, there will be no reason you can't achieve anything you desire.

Tyler and I balance each other out very well. I entered this relationship as a creative, free-spirited thinker, while he is more of a logical, analytical person. We've influenced each other in ways that allow us to blend our contrasting qualities, allowing us to confidently make significant decisions that consistently work out in our favor. And when our decisions lead to unexpected detours, we've learned to view those as valuable lessons. If you can approach life this way, there are no wrong decisions, no missteps, and no accidents—everything simply is.

11

LESSONS IN SILENCE

On top of people being coerced into being something they're not, there seems to be this entitlement that comes along with that. Nowadays, everyone has developed this *need to be right*. We live in a world where so many people feel the need to express their opinions so wholeheartedly that families get torn apart over differing beliefs. In needing the last word, bridges get burned. A huge takeaway from my life experience has been about keeping my mouth shut. There's a time and a place for everything but most of the time, taking a second to think before we immaturely blurt out our thoughts is a wise choice to make. The majority of the hostility that many people express stems from that need to be right. I've been a part of that cycle, and trust me, it does everything but benefit growth. We are all experiencing reality differently, so it's impossible for any two of us to see the world the same. So, if you're seeing life through your own lens and I'm seeing it through mine, how can it possibly make sense for us to argue when we're living entirely different lives in completely separate realities? It can't! So, before you allow yourself to get triggered by someone or something, catch and remind yourself of this very concept. It really puts into perspective how every argument can be avoided, nullifying that need to be right.

There will be times when you won't remember this, and you'll find yourself heated in the middle of an argument. This happens all the time in my life, and when I reflect back to each encounter, I try to see where I lost control of keeping my composure. When I am conscious of how I respond to people, I'm easily guided to remember to be silent unless a response is needed. I remind myself not to take things too personally, and to not let my emotions grab hold of the conversation. This is a practice we will all be refining for the rest of our lives, taking a moment of pause before responding. As I've already mentioned, there will be many tests that pop up for you in your daily life; a person who's ready to argue being one of them. You always have the choice of engaging in that argument or taking a step back and redirecting it altogether. You'll notice you'll have some type of choice in *all* situations. Always choose to be quiet first, and then respond. An example of this is the fact that I've been relatively quiet for the past few years as I learn to navigate this new perception and new life, while I simultaneously process the things I've been through without professional help—my response is this book.

Aside from taking an extra second to respond to the

external, there is so much that can be learned from silence as a whole. A societal norm we've all fallen victim to is always needing to fill the silence with *something*. Whether that be music, gossip, or surface-level small talk; at some point in our conversations we've had a second of silence that made us feel uncomfortable. We've coined the term "awkward silence," and we judge people based on if their silent moments make us feel weird or not. But what if we chose to see that silence as a powerful tool to help us stay anchored in the moment? An old friend of mine had visited me after a lot of time had passed, and we had much to catch up on. Instead of jumping right into every detail of everything that's happened since the last time we saw each other, we were able to slow down the conversation and let it flow naturally with lots of silence in between. We gave each other a chance to take in our surroundings and be with ourselves while simultaneously sharing space with each other. We've become accustomed to always feeling the need to speak, and in doing so, we often neglect the vital aspect of simply being. This constant need to express ourselves can disconnect us from our true selves, as we become overwhelmed by distractions and the unspoken expectation to always have something to contribute. By prioritizing conversation over reflection, or neglecting balancing both simultaneously, we risk losing touch with our inner world, which is essential for genuine connection with ourselves and others. If you have a consciously created response, let it flow. Yet, if you're speaking out of obligation, you will eventually find yourself drained of energy. Embracing silence begins with sitting with yourself first. This process highlights the pattern of personal growth: When you become comfortable in your own skin, mind, and heart, you can carry that sense of contentment into all of your interactions. See how full circle "the work" is?

12

MEDITATION MAKES A DIFFERENCE

If you've been avoiding self-reflection for most of your life, meditation may feel challenging at first. But if you commit to practicing consistently for a few weeks, you'll uncover insights about yourself that you never realized were there. Find a quiet and safe place to sit, close your eyes, and follow your breath. It's really that simple. With every breath you breathe in, follow that up with a long exhalation, allowing yourself to breathe at a pace that's comfortable and doesn't feel forced. If this is new to you, only focus on following your breath (meaning only permit your attention to focus on your breathing). If you find your mind racing with thoughts, redirect your focus back to your breath. There's no need for a specific goal, just immerse yourself fully in the rhythm of your breathing. Start with a few minutes each day, slowly lengthening the time as you become more comfortable. Try making this a regular practice, carving out dedicated moments for yourself each day.

Meditation can take many forms, and it's important to realize that not everyone can sit still right away. Sometimes, especially for me, this can lead to increased agitation. If that's true for you too, consider engaging in an active practice that allows you to focus completely. When I feel anxious or wake up out of sorts, sitting still can be more counterproductive than beneficial. My insides feel like I'm buzzing, and my limbs feel like they need to move. The more I ignore those feelings and attempt to force a still meditation, the stronger my frustration becomes. Explore movement as a way to channel that energy if this is the case for you. When I have days like this, I'll either go for a really long walk or I'll go to the gym and lift weights to move around the stuck energy. I've never left the gym feeling worse than when I got there. Movement of any kind can be meditative as long as you are giving all of your attention to whatever you're doing as well as remembering to breathe. Once you've found a way to release pent-up energy, returning to a stationary meditation will become easier to tolerate. This transition will take time, so don't force it if it doesn't feel right.

Finding time to meditate can be challenging, especially in the midst of a busy life, but that shouldn't deter you from practicing at all. Even a few minutes can be effective, whether it's during your kids' naps, right after you wake up, just before bed, or during a brief break at work. There's always room to breathe. If you can find time to scroll through your phone or watch TV, you can find time to meditate. Stay accountable and disciplined in prioritizing this practice for yourself.

13

THE POWER OF DISCIPLINE

Being disciplined and having self-control ultimately paves the way for personal growth and a deeper sense of purpose. Be disciplined in your thoughts and actions and have self-control over what you allow your mind to partake in. This means consciously choosing what you engage in, in every sense. When you practice self-control, you empower yourself to resist fleeting temptations that can derail the progress you're working toward. For example:

Men—if you're in a relationship, stop giving other people of interest your attention. This is a very simple concept. If you're serious about being with someone, they deserve your full focus. If this is hard for you, you shouldn't be in that relationship and clearly have a lot of work to do in regard to your discipline.

Women—if you're in a relationship and you want your significant other to be dedicated to you, you too need to stop making yourself available to other people of interest. It's a two-way street and needs to be worked on together. You both need to set boundaries as needed. Have the self-control and the discipline to give your partner the respect they deserve.

This concept of self-discipline and respect goes way

beyond relationships and equally applies to yourself. Most of us, if not all, set goals we strive to achieve. It's up to you and only you to be disciplined enough to take proper action and steps required to achieve those desired goals. I've been able to adopt a mindset where if I want something bad enough, I'm going to do what it takes in order to get it. Being sick for so long when I was constantly giving attention to what I put in and on my body was a giant slap in the face; through years of pain and frustration, I never gave up trying to achieve better health. In doing that, I was able to become many different versions of myself, each being better than the last. I was persistent, and even though it took a really long time to level out, I became healthy enough to grow a child inside of me—my biggest accomplishment. And since my daughter has been born, I've dedicated my life to making sure I'm always working on improving myself as a person and staying healthy so that I can be an example for her to look up to. That means taking care of my mind first, and everything else will follow.

I've learned in just the short 18 months of being a mother so far that being a parent takes a lot of discipline. My daughter knows exactly which buttons to push that trigger the things in me that need the most attention. And because I want to be better and I want to continue to improve, I have a choice to make in those moments: allow myself to be overtaken by emotion and react in a similar way I have been treated in the past, or choose to slow down and not allow my emotions to control my words or actions, choosing to be better. I do my best to be as understanding and patient with my daughter as I can, which takes a hell of a lot of self-control for someone who grew up being a walking landmine. If you choose to have children, it's the most rewarding but challenging endeavor you could ever take on. But even in knowing that, if you can stay dedicated to your self-work, stay disciplined and have a good sense of self-control, you'll make leaps and bounds in your progress as a human.

Relationships also challenge your discipline at its very core. My husband knows precisely what triggers my "landmine" moments, and I equally understand how to reciprocate. We both have an understanding that part of choosing to be in a relationship (especially for 14 plus years so far) is accepting that the other person is there *specifically* to test your triggers- to push your buttons, to get you to that boiling point. On the other side of that boiling point is where change and growth can truly take place. So, even though it's one of the hardest things to control in the moment, if you and your significant other find yourselves in an argument, try to remember that this moment is an opportunity for growth. It reveals aspects of yourself and your partner that may need attention and understanding. Embrace the conflict as a chance to explore deeper feelings rather than seeing the situation as "just another fight". (This is much easier said than done so, yet again, it's another aspect to be patient with yourself with!)

To sum this up, the journey of personal growth, self-discipline, and respect within relationships is an ongoing process that requires dedication and intentionality. Whether in romantic partnerships or as individuals, the challenges we face serve as catalysts for profound understanding and transformation. Each moment of conflict offers a chance to reflect, learn, and evolve—both for ourselves and those we love. By embracing these opportunities, we not only strengthen our connections but also cultivate the resilience necessary for personal achievement. As we navigate the nuances of relationships, with others and with ourselves, remember that discipline and self-control are not just tools for managing external challenges; they are essential for tending to our inner world. By doing this, we set an example for those around us, especially our children, solidifying that growth and self-improvement are indeed lifelong commitments. The journey toward becoming the best version of ourselves is as rewarding as it is challenging—an adventure worth every effort.

14

THE LAST BREATH

Death is the root of all of our fears. We keep ourselves healthy and safe the best we can, so we don't die. We are overprotective of our children, so they don't die. We would never approach a lion in the wild because we don't want it to eat us, so we don't die. We would never willingly jump out of a plane without a parachute because we don't want to die. It's human instinct to stay alive. Somewhere down the line that deep instinctual need to live got translated to being *afraid* of dying. Children are perceived as having no fear because they're closest to the source of where we all come from; they instinctually know not to fear. I believe fear is learned. I can't recall ever holding the fear of dying as a child, but as I got older and experienced more life, that fear definitely snuck in. It's still not clear to me whether I developed a fear of dying itself or if I developed a fear of losing the people and experiences of the life I've worked so hard to be conscious of. I've teetered on the brink of death quite a few times in my life, and because of the culmination of my experiences, I can confidently say that we have absolutely nothing to fear.

Whether or not my theory of me actually dying after my

first seizure is true, *something* happened when I came out of my body and rose to the top of my shower. Although I cannot explain exactly where I went, I was *somewhere*. My awareness didn't just "go dark." I found myself in a space of pure contentment, painless bliss, objectively watching tragic events transpire below me. I felt supported by a force I could not physically see, and I felt safe as if threats didn't exist. I had no emotional attachment to seeing my own body seizing on the floor of the tub or seeing the fear emanating from my mother and mother-in-law when they found me. I, and everything occurring in that moment, just *was*.

I now walk through life with way less fear than I used to, and that's not to be taken as "I'm better than you", it's to further exemplify that it is possible to simply **exist** with no strings attached. I may get sucked into the drama of events playing out around me from time to time, but at the end of the day I'll usually come back to self and realize that it's just yet another thing *happening*. If you can get to a point of existing where you can feel and let go simultaneously of the emotional attachments that are presented to us, you'll become more content in your humanness. Oftentimes, my non-reaction to situations that would cause someone else to cry or become angry, comes off as I just don't care. And although my sarcastic personality would like to agree, that just isn't true. I am able to feel the emotions that will come up for me, and then quickly switch to seeing through the situation for what it is and what it's trying to teach me. Maybe that's just me, maybe I'm just the heartless bitch I've been pinned on being in the past, or maybe it's just an unhealthy way to process; regardless, I view being able to dissect tough situations in this way as a superpower. It can be painful, but it also can be beautiful to allow what is, to be.

If you are someone who's terrified of death, where the thought of it scares you to the point of not being able to even ponder it, I hope my experience has sparked an interest in you to further explore. No matter what you believe in— whether religious, atheist, or undecided altogether on the matter—there is no reason to fear death. It's fun to keep in mind that your perception will be your outcome. I personally believe that something more happens when we die, so I experienced a situation where that stood true because that was my wholehearted belief. What you think, what you believe, and what you stick to will be your reality when that time comes. Do with that information what you will. When you can live each day without fear standing in the way, you've successfully become resilient. Take that resilience and pass it along, never stop reminding others that they, too, have the ability to achieve the same.

15

A BEAUTIFUL STORM: FINAL WORDS

Put aside the physical and emotional pain, the many versions of myself that have died before my own eyes; overlook the rough childhood experiences, the doubt and shame, and the cruel words that shot arrows through my heart. Ignore the loss of self I've experienced on more than one occasion; disregard the heartache from having soccer torn from my life, the arguments, the fights, and the anxiety. Set aside the friends I've lost because of the way I've changed due to my circumstances, the pressure to hold my family together growing up, the lonely nights spent pondering leaving this world, the attempts, the struggles— and you know what's still here? Me. I'm still here. I'm still fighting for my life each day I open my eyes. Some days are harder than others, but I won't give up. I deserve to be here. And so do you.

There are parts of me that still haven't fully adjusted to this new reality, and I know that by the time I feel fully settled, I'll be in the midst of another transition to an even newer reality. I used to be so confident in myself as a whole, in my relationship, and in my writing. But after my last experience with my health, life and everyone and everything in it still feel so foreign, even years later. But as I've attempted to settle into this current version of myself, those things have all greatly improved and will continue to improve the more I let things be. The fear of being rejected by others, the fear of not being enough for my husband, or enough for my daughter, and the fear of being harshly criticized for the blunt way that I speak, think, and write still creep in; but slowly and steadily, life is starting to become clearer.

Tyler's been on me about finishing this book. My argument was that this part of my life was over and is now old news; this world is too fast paced to dwell on anything for more than a few days. I'd say how I didn't think anyone would care to hear what I've really gone through because, clearly, we all go through something—many somethings. Why should my story be so lucky to be known? Why would anyone care to hear me vent of my struggles? Or to hear me applaud myself for getting through it without giving up? I don't want the attention, or the applause. My struggles have only been for me to experience as well as the lessons I signed up to conquer in this life. Very few have been lucky enough to be a part of my web of growth, and to those who know who they are—I deeply admire that you've stayed by my side when you certainly didn't have to in such excruciating

156

conditions.

As the reader, you have many choices to make. You can sit here and say, 'I know all,' or you can sit here and say, 'I know nothing.' Both options have their own consequences. *Knowing all* will close you off to all that is yet to be. *Knowing nothing* will allow for an infinite amount of knowledge to be accessible to those who seek it. The choice is yours. Love, be, and live free. If you've read this far, I deeply thank you for taking the time to voluntarily dive into my world for a brief time. I'm sure you're extremely excited to get back to your own world with your own melodramas playing out. But I'd like to leave you with this last bit:

No matter what you're going through, no matter how fucked up your situation seems, no matter how much pain you're enduring—whether physically, mentally, or emotionally—no matter what is going on in your life right now, **you are alive**. Being alive is the greatest gift you could ever receive. You'll have terrible days, and you'll have amazing ones, all while having dense ones in between the extremes. Regardless of what kind of day you have, you were gifted with the day. When you're riding that low wave, remember to turn inward because you're the only one who has somewhat control over your reactions to your experiences, and your reactions are what shapes the reality in front of you. Do your best to recognize the slightest positive changes in your mindset and how you handle situations. You are never stuck, you are never not loved, you are never not enough, and most importantly, you are never alone. You are constantly improving as a conscious being. Be proud of where you've gotten yourself to. All is how it's supposed to be, always—it couldn't be any other way, or else you wouldn't exist.

It's at this time that I truly understand that I know nothing. I'm a vessel for experience and information gained through those experiences. There have been many phases of Hailey who thought she had all the answers, but I am so grateful to be free from those previous versions of her. Right here, right now, I know nothing. After the flare in 2021 when I got to Hawaii, I arrived with the clearest, emptiest mind I ever had. Whether or not that was the start of the comedown from psychosis or the medications, regardless, I still for a brief moment felt what it feels like to be mentally free. Parts of that have carried over into my everyday life currently, and at times it makes it exceedingly difficult to engage in meaningless conversations, or just conversation in general. Somewhere down the long, crooked road of hell that I crawled through, I chose to be the observer. And that position has been what I've chosen to settle into because of the challenges it presents. It's so difficult to observe without judging or without having to put in my two cents. For so long, I've always had to be heard and if I wasn't, I'd get loud or I'd get defensive. But through my struggles I've finally found life's greatest test for me: shut up and sit in the silence. I invite you to do the same, or at least give it a try despite its difficulty.

To some, none of the ramblings in this book will make sense to the thinking mind. And that's okay; it doesn't have to—because the point of this book isn't to tell you the right ways to live, be, or think. The point of this book is to open up avenues of thought, to broaden your awareness, and to help you construct your own individual ways of existing. To have you read between the words and the pauses to find the deeper meaning of what realizations my experiences have brought me, and to see how they can benefit you. To prove that there's way more than one way to exist. And, most importantly, to shed light on a subject often overlooked: death.

I could have continued with this book, adding in each and every lesson I've learned, but due to the nature of simplicity, it would have been vastly repetitive. Why complicate things that were meant to be simple? Everything I've said could be false, or from the mind of the distorted reality I experienced, but for me, whoever that is in this moment—it's all true. Most people spend their entire lives searching for their purpose. Through my trials and tribulations, I've come to realize that my purpose is quite simple: to be; to be a mother, to be a wife, to be an energy that can't be destroyed, to be an inspiration, to be resilience itself. In a storm, there are both beauty and disaster—I am both, and that's okay with me. I understand that I'm human. But I also understand that there are parts of me that are not human. If there's good in me, it's only right that there's bad as well. There's real evil that exists within me, in all of us. A monster waiting to be acknowledged. Some of us bury that monster so far down, pushing it off to deal with in a future lifetime, carrying around a deep pain that can't quite be reached. And then there are those of us who are up next in line. The ones who are here to face all of our most demanding demons, to befriend them, to really learn what it's like to release them. The beast that lives in me had her time to shine, and shine she did, destroying anyone and anything that was in her path, including herself. But now she knows who's in charge, and she'll stay tame as long as I allow her to exist and not push her away. The next lesson I've learned, that I'll finish off this life with, is learning when to utilize her power and when not to. Like the Hulk, we coexist as one now. All is meant to be.

Thank you for reading and thank you for being. If your heart's beating, keep going. Be better, live better, and free yourself from your own self-inflicted prison. From the depths of the interstices of my reality to the space I'm in now and the spaces I'll go, namaste.

A vitally important parting reminder; *Memento Mori.*

"Soon you will be dead and none of it will matter."

– Marcus Aurelius, *Meditations: A New Translation*

www.ingramcontent.com/pod-product-compliance
Lightning Source LLC
LaVergne TN
LVHW041320080426
835513LV00008B/524